Notes on Antimicrobial Th

Notes on Antimicrobial Therapy

Jane Symonds
MB ChB MRCPath
Consultant Microbiologist, Dudley Health
Authority, Dudley, West Midlands;
Honorary Clinical Lecturer, Department of
Medical Microbiology, University of
Birmingham

Foreword by
D S Reeves
MB MRCPath
Consultant Medical Microbiologist,
Department of Medical Microbiology,
Southmead Hospital, Bristol

CHURCHILL LIVINGSTONE
EDINBURGH LONDON MELBOURNE AND NEW YORK 1983

CHURCHILL LIVINGSTONE
Medical Division of Longman Group Limited

Distributed in the United States of America by
Churchill Livingstone Inc., 1560 Broadway, New York,
N.Y. 10036, and by associated companies, branches and
representatives throughout the world.

First published 1983

ISBN 0 443 02953 9

British Library Cataloguing in Publication Data
Symonds, Jane
    Notes on antimicrobial therapy.—
    (Churchill Livingstone medical text)
    1. Antibiotics
    I. Title
    615' 329   RM267

Library of Congress Cataloging in Publication Data
Symonds, Jane, 1948–
    Notes on antimicrobial therapy.
    (Churchill Livingstone medical text)
    Includes index.
    1. Anti-infective agents. 2. Communicable
diseases—
Chemotherapy. I. Title. II. Series. [DNLM:
1. Antibiotics—Therapeutic use. QV 350 S988n]
RM262.S95   1983   616.9'061   83–5159

Printed in Singapore by
The Print House (Pte) Ltd

Foreword

Infection is a frequent primary or complicating illness in all types of patient. Because antibiotics have low toxicity relative to most other drugs they are prescribed by virtually all clinicians, often with little thought as to their proper use. The usual fault is inappropriate prescribing rather than the more serious one, for the individual patient, of failure to give therapy at all. Nevertheless, to receive either an antibiotic unnecessarily or the wrong agent can result in individual harm due to the occurrence of avoidable toxicity or failure to control infection. In community terms poor prescribing can be an added financial drain on an already stretched health service and, ultimately far more alarmingly, encourage the ever present progression of bacterial resistance, a phenomenon which might well not be readily reversed in the future by more restrained prescribing.

Antibiotic therapy is everyone's prerogative and almost nobody's pride and is often taught poorly to students as a consequence. The publication of this excellent small book by Dr Symonds is thus most welcome, aiming as it does to give the essentials of antibiotic therapy for students and the non-expert prescriber. Diligently read by students and conscientiously used by house officers it must result in the better use of one of the most abused groups of drugs to the benefit of the infected patient and of the population at large. The inclusion of the less frequently prescribed antiviral and antihelmintic agents is a bonus in that information on their use is widely dispersed.

Bristol, 1983   D.S. Reeves

Preface

Antibiotics are amongst the most widely prescribed drugs both in hospital and community practice. Medical students are expected to become familiar with a large and ever expanding group of agents whose proper application demands an understanding not only of the antibacterial properties of individual agents but also of their pharmacology, toxicology and of the impact of extensive use on microbial ecology, (not to mention cost).

This book is intended to outline in perspective the drugs most widely used in treatment of infection in medical practice today. It is written primarily for medical students, but practical details such as dosages have been included so that it can also be used by practising physicians, who may refer to it as a summary of current antimicrobial therapy.

I am grateful to Dr David Reeves for offering most helpful advice during the preparation of this book, and for writing its foreword. I am much indebted to Dr Richard Wise for sustained help and encouragement, and to Dr Peter Brown who first suggested the idea of this book. My sincere thanks also to Mrs Dorothy Hammond for invaluable secretarial help.

Dudley, 1983   J.S.

Contents

1. The development of antimicrobial therapy   1
2. Modes of action of antimicrobial agents   3
3. Antibiotic treatment of infections caused by human
   pathogens   6
4. Bacterial resistance to antibiotics   14
5. Strategies in the management of infection   18
6. Antibiotics in combination   21
7. Properties and use of antimicrobial agents   23
   The penicillins   23
   The cephalosporins   34
   The aminoglycosides   41
   Macrolides and lincosamides   45
   Sodium fusidate   47
   Polymixins   48
   The sulphonamides, co-trimoxazole, trimethoprim   49
   Chloramphenicol   53
   Tetracyclines   54
   Other antibacterial drugs (vancomycin, metronidazole)   57
   Urinary antimicrobials   59
8. Antituberculous drugs   62
9. Antifungal agents   68
10. Antiprotozoal agents   74
11. Antihelmintics   82
12. Antibiotic prophylaxis   84
13. Laboratory control of antimicrobial therapy   89
14. Antibiotic use in renal and hepatic failure   92
15. Antiviral chemotherapy   97
16. Antibiotic policies   99
Further reading   102
Index   103

1

The development of antimicrobial therapy

Empirical antimicrobial therapy has probably been practised for centuries—the annointing of septic wounds with poultices of mouldy bread (quite possibly rich in antibiotic-producing fungi) is chronicled in some of the earliest accounts of traditional medicine.

SYNTHETIC ANTIBACTERIAL AGENTS

Paul Ehrlich is regarded as the founder of modern antimicrobial therapy, and was the first to seek the 'magic bullet' or substance that would destroy microbes without harming human tissue. Working in Germany in the first decade of this century, he discovered that the dye trypan red cured experimental trypanosomiasis in mice; he also studied the activity of the arsenical Salvarsan on *Treponema pallidum*. Much research interest focussed subsequently on dyes, but it was not until 1935 that Domagk reported the activity of the dye Prontosil against streptococci, not only in experimental mice but also in the treatment of his own daughter, who recovered dramatically from serious streptococcal sepsis in response to Prontosil. Prontosil itself is bacteriologically inactive but is converted in the body to sulphanilamide (the first sulphonamide). Sulphonamides were of enormous value in controlling streptococcal sepsis, pneumococcal pneumonia and gonorrhoea until widespread emergence of resistance in the 1940s considerably limited their effectiveness.

Other synthetic agents developed subsequently include isoniazid for treatment of tuberculosis, and the nitroimidazoles (e.g. metronidazole) for infections caused by anaerobic bacteria and protozoa.

NATURALLY-OCCURRING ANTIBIOTICS

Alexander Fleming is popularly recognised as the first to have made scientific observations on the antibacterial properties of fungi. In 1929 he observed inhibition of staphylococci on culture medium contaminated by the mould *Penicillium*. However, he was unable to

1

extract or stabilise enough of the active principle to perform any extensive tests of its effectiveness in therapy. It was not until 1940 that Florey & Chain, having developed a technique for purification of a stable form of penicillin, were able to report studies of its therapeutic activity.

Searches for other naturally-occurring antibiotics have yielded griseofulvin (1939), streptomycin (1944), chloramphenicol (1947), tetracycline (1948), cephalosporin C (1948), erythromycin (1952), rifampicin (1957), fusidic acid (1960), lincomycin (1962) and gentamicin (1963) among many others. Some, such as chloramphenicol, can now be produced entirely synthetically and others, including the cephalosporins and penicillins, have been modified chemically to yield semi-synthetic compounds with improved antimicrobial and pharmacological properties. So great is the choice of antimicrobial drugs now available that rational prescribing is becoming increasingly complex. Nevertheless, individual prescribers will usually need only a limited number of antibiotics with which to gain experience and confidence.

2

Modes of action of antimicrobial agents

An ideal antimicrobial agent should act selectively against bacteria, interfering with microbial metabolism whilst having little or no effect on human cells.

There are four principle target sites for antibacterial activity:

1. The cell wall
2. The cell membrane
3. Nucleic acids
4. Protein synthesis

1. ANTIBACTERIAL AGENTS WHICH INTERFERE WITH CELL WALL SYNTHESIS

Bacteria differ from mammalian cells in having rigid cell walls. Penicillins and cephalosporins inhibit synthesis of bacterial cell walls but have little or no effect on human tissue. Bacterial stability depends on polypepetide links which unite layers of glycan forming the cell wall, a process interrupted by penicillins and cephalosporins. Deprived of external support, bacterial cells rupture. Penicillin is active mainly against Gram-positive bacteria; it is unable penetrate the thicker walls of Gram-negative coliform organisms although neisseria species (Gram-negative cocci) are susceptible. Broad-spectrum penicillins (such as ampicillin) and the cephalosporins are active against both Gram-positive and Gram-negative species.

Beta-lactamase enzymes which destroy penicillins account for penicillin-resistance in 80 to 90% of strains of *Staphylococcus aureus* in hospitals. Other beta-lactamases produced by Gram-negative bacteria are responsible for resistance to ampicillin and cephalosporins. These enzymes are so-called because they cleave the beta-lactam ring of the penicillin or cephalosporin nucleus, rendering the drug microbiologically inactive. Beta-lactamases are found just within the cell wall and remain closely associated with the cell in Gram-negative bacilli; staphylococci, however, liberate penicillinase into their

3

environment, and may be responsible for failure of penicillin to eradicate sensitive organisms such as streptococci when both streptococci and staphylococci are present, in skin infections for example.

Vancomycin, cycloserine and bacitracin also act by inhibiting cell wall synthesis, (but at a different stage of peptidoglycan formation to that attacked by penicillins or cephalosporins). They are not affected by beta-lactamases.

2. ANTIBIOTICS WHICH INTERFERE WITH CELL MEMBRANE FUNCTION

The cell membrane controls passage of molecules and ions into and out of the cell. Polymixins attach to the cell membrane, modifying its control over the passage of ions and causing lysis of the cell.

3. ANTIBACTERIAL AGENTS WHICH INTERFERE WITH NUCLEIC ACID SYNTHESIS

a. Nalidixic acid and rifampicin prevent replication of nucleic acids in bacteria, so that protein synthesis stops.

b. Metronidazole is active against bacteria and protozoa which grow only in the absence of air (anaerobes); these organisms reduce the drug to its 2-hydroxy-metabolite, which causes bacterial DNA to fragment.

c. Sulphonamides and trimethoprim interfere with synthesis of folic acid, an essential co-factor in nucleotide synthesis. Both drugs act on sequential steps of the same metabolic pathway and their combined action has been said to be synergistic. Sulphonamides inhibit dihydrofolate synthetase, which catalyses conversion of para-amino-benzoic acid (a structural analogue of sulphonamides) to dihydrofolate, as the first step in folate synthesis. Dihydrofolate is then converted to tetrahydrofolate by the enzyme dihydrofolate reductase, whose activity is inhibited by trimethoprim. Human cells use dietary folic or folinic acid for nucleotide synthesis, so that normal doses of folate antagonists infrequently lead to folate depletion (except when demand is increased, as in pregnancy, or when folate is lacking in the diet). Enzymes responsible for folate synthesis in humans are much less sensitive to sulphonamides and trimethoprim than bacterial enzymes. Protozoal cells however are susceptible to folate antagonists; for example pyrimethamine has antimalarial activity, and co-trimoxazole is active against Pneumocystis carini.

Sulphonamide resistance is often due to the emergence of mutant organisms whose dihydrofolate synthetase has reduced affinity for sulphonamides. In other strains it is due to production of excess para-aminobenzoic acid, which enables the organisms to continue to generate folic acid. Resistance to trimethoprim is usually a result of reduced affinity of dihydrofolate reductase for trimethoprim.

4. ANTIBACTERIAL AGENTS WHICH INTERFERE WITH PROTEIN SYNTHESIS

Bacterial proteins are assembled from amino acids on ribosomes consisting of 30S and 50S subunits. These differ from ribosomes of mammalian cells, which are not susceptible to agents capable of disturbing bacterial ribosome function.

RNA is responsible for building up amino acids into polypeptide chains, according to sequences specified by the DNA code.

a. Aminoglycosides prevent protein synthesis by binding to 30S ribosome subunits. This causes the RNA code to be misread, and inappropriate amino acids are incorporated into the peptide chain, forming faulty proteins. Resistance to aminoglycosides arises when bacteria produce inactivating enzymes (adenylases, acetylases and phosphotransferases) which may modify the structure of the drug so that it is unable to penetrate the cell.

b. Tetracycline and chloramphenicol interfere with attachment of amino acids to the ribosome, interrupting protein synthesis. Growth in vitro usually resumes when these drugs are withdrawn, so that they are bacteristatic, rather than bactericidal in action i.e. they only arrest growth, but do not kill (see p. 21). Resistant mutants arise fairly readily, since only minor molecular changes render bacteria insensitive to these drugs; resistance to chloramphenicol in some bacteria is also due to enzyme inactivation (see p. 15).

c. Erythromycin binds to the 50S subunit of the ribosome at a site also bound by clindamycin; cross-resistance is shown by some bacteria to these two agents.

d. Fusidic acid also interferes with attachment of amino acids at the ribosome and protein synthesis ceases. Resistance emerges readily in bacteria exposed to fusidic acid because of selection of resistant mutants.

Erythromycin, clindamycin and fusidic acid are active against Gram-positive organisms but not against Gram-negative aerobic bacilli because of their inability to penetrate the outer lipopolysaccharide component of the Gram-negative cell wall.

3

Antibiotic treatment of infections caused by human pathogens

Tables 3.1, 3.2 and 3.3 summarise the antibiotic treatment of human infections. It is important that management of patients with difficult or unusual infections should involve close co-operation between clinician and microbiologist.

Table 3.1 Summary of antibiotic treatment of human pathogens

Organism	Urinary tract	Upper respiratory tract	Lower respiratory tract	Soft tissue	Septicaemia Endocarditis*	Meningitis	Bone joint	Other	Comments
Gram-positive cocci *Staphylococcus aureus*			1. Flucloxacillin + fusidic acid 2. Clindamycin	1. Flucloxacillin 2. Erythromycin or cephalosporin	1. Flucloxacillin (+ fusidic acid for deep-seated sepsis) 2. Clindamycin or vancomycin 3. Erythromycin for less serious infection	Usually post-traumatic: flucloxacillin + rifampicin	1. Flucloxacillin + fusidic acid 2. Clindamycin or cephalosporin (eg cefazolin or cefuroxime)		1. Penicillin is preferred to flucloxacillin in treatment of penicillin-sensitive staphylococci 2. Activity of flucloxacillin may be limited in some sites because of its high degree of protein-binding (∴ fusidic acid may be included as an adjuvant) 3. Clindamycin should be reserved for serious deep-seated infection because of its potential toxicity (colitis).
Beta-haemolytic streptococci		1. Penicillin 2. Erythromycin	1. Benzylpenicillin 2. Cefuroxime	1. Penicillin 2. Erythromycin	1. Benzylpenicillin *(+ gentamicin for endocarditis) 2. Cefuroxime	Group B. streptococcal infection in neonates 1. Benzyl penicillin + gentamicin 2. Chloramphenicol			Penicillin is required in high dosage at 4 hourly intervals for serious infections. Probenecid may be given to delay excretion.
Strept. pneumoniae		1. Penicillin 2. Erythromycin	1. Benzylpenicillin 2. erythromycin		1. Penicillin 2. Cefuroxime	1. Benzyl penicillin 2. Chloramphenicol			

Table 3.1 (Cont'd)

Organism	Urinary tract	Upper respiratory tract	Lower respiratory tract	Soft tissue	Septicaemia Endocarditis*	Meningitis	Bone joint	Other	Comments
Alpha-haemolytic & non-haemolytic streptococci ('viridans' streptococci)			e.g. pneumonia caused by Strept. milleri 1. Benzylpenicillin 2. Erythromycin	e.g. abscesses caused by Strept. milleri 1. Benzylpenicillin 2. Erythromycin, (usually as adjunct to drainage)	*Endocarditis 1. Benzyl penicillin (+ gentamicin initially for most cases) 2. Cefuroxime				In endocarditis addition of gentamicin to penicillin produces a more rapidly cidal effect than penicillin alone. Oral amoxycillin may be used subsequently if response is good.
Strept. faecalis	Ampicillin				*Endocarditis 1. Benzyl penicillin or ampicillin + gentamicin. 2. Vancomycin				Always monitor bactericidal activity of serum of patients treated for endocarditis to ensure that therapy is adequate (discuss with microbiologist)
Gram-positive bacilli Corynebacterium diphtheriae		1. Benzylpenicillin 2. Erythromycin							1. Early treatment with antitoxin essential 2. Carriers should be treated with erythromycin
Listeria monocytogenes			Benzylpenicillin	Benzylpenicillin	Ampicillin	Ampicillin (+ gentamicin)			
Bacillus anthracis Branching filamentous bacteria: Actinomyces israeli								Benzylpenicillin initially, continuing oral treatment with amoxycillin	Courses of at least 6 weeks required

Organism					Notes
asteroides					
Gram-negative cocci: *Neisseria meningitidis*			Benzylpenicillin	1. Benzylpenicillin 2. Chloramphenicol	Very close contacts e.g. household members should be given prophylaxis (see p. 85)
Neisseria gonorrhoeae				1. Benzylpenicillin 2. Doxycycline or cotrimoxazole	Neonatal ophthalmia should be treated with penicillin eye drops, with systemic penicillin if necessary
Gram-negative bacilli: *Haemophilus influenzae*	(i) Sinusitis, middle ear infection or pharyngitis: ampicillin or co-trimoxazole or trimethoprim (ii) Epiglottitis (usually in young children): ampicillin (if sensitive) or chloramphenicol	(i) Bronchitis: ampicillin or co-trimoxazole or trimethoprim (ii) Pneumonia: ampicillin or co-trimoxazole or cefuroxime.	Ampicillin (if sensitive) or chloramphenicol	Ampicillin	In the UK the incidence of ampicillin resistance in capsulated *H. influenzae* is about 10%. ∴ chloramphenicol is probably the treatment of choice initially for serious infection
Bordetella pertussis	Erythromycin	Chloramphenicol for severe *B. pertussis* pneumonia in young children			Antibiotics must be started as soon as possible if they are to influence the course of the illness. They probably have little effect on established infection.

Table 3.1 (Cont'd)

Organism	Urinary tract	Upper respiratory tract	Lower respiratory tract	Soft tissue	Septicaemia Endocarditis*	Meningitis	Bone-joint	Other	Comments
Brucella spp								Tetracycline or co-trimoxazole	Continue treatment for 6–8 weeks
'Coliform' bacilli: (i) *Esch. coli*	1. Trimethoprim or co-trimoxazole 2. Nitrofurantoin (not for upper urinary tract infections) NB: ampicillin is preferred if strains are sensitive but 30% are resistant				1. Gentamicin (*+ mezlocillin for endocarditis) 2. Cefotaxime/ cefuroxime	Neonatal meningitis: gentamicin and mezlocillin, or chloramphenicol			Antibiotic sensitivity tests give best guide to therapy since sensitivities are not always predictable (although most coliforms are susceptible to gentamicin).
Klebsiella spp	1. Cephalexin 2. Trimethoprim or co-trimoxazole 3. Cephalosporin				1. Gentamicin 2. Cefotaxime/ cefuroxime	as for E. coli			
Proteus spp	1. Most strains (i.e. *Pr. mirabilis*) are sensitive to ampicillin 2. Co-trimoxazole or trimethoprim				1. Gentamicin (*+ mezlocillin for endocarditis) 2. Cefotaxime or cefuroxime	as for E. coli			
Enterobacter Serratia Providencia					Gentamicin,				Often resistant to antibiotics ∴ therapy should be guided by labora-

Organism			
	tobramycin; carfecillin if oral treatment is required	azlocillin or pip-era-cillin	more active than gentamicin against *Ps. aeruginosa* and is preferred for deep sepsis
	tobramycin. *For endocarditis (eg drug addicts) use tobramycin + azlocillin		
Salmonella typhi		Co-trimoxazole. Chloramphenicol is used for severe infection	Chemotherapy only required for systemic infections — co-trimoxazole
Other Salmonellae food poisoning (serotypes)			Gastro-enteritis is usually self limiting
Shigella spp			*S. sonnei* diarrhoea is usually self-limiting; other species may require antibiotic treatment. Choice of antibiotic is required for severe disease must be determined by sensitivity tests
Other Gram-negative organisms *Vibrio cholerae*			1. Tetracycline 2. Co-trimoxazole. Fluid replacement and electrolyte balance important
Campylobacter			Gastro-enteritis usually self-limiting. If treatment required, give erthromycin; or gentamicin for serious systemic infection
Legionella	Erythromycin in high doses. Rifampicin may be added if response is poor		

Table 3.2 Antimicrobial treatment of infections caused by anaerobic bacteria

Organism	Infection	Antibiotic treatment 1. 1st choice 2. Alternative(s)
Clostridia: *Cl. botulinum*	Botulism	1. Benzylpenicillin to prevent production of more toxin. NB: early administration of antitoxin is most important.
Cl. tetani	Tetanus	1. Benzylpenicillin. NB: early administration of antitoxin and removal of devitalised tissue are more important. Penicillin has no activity against spores or pre-formed toxin. 2. Metronidazole.
Cl. perfringens	Gas gangrene	1. Benzylpenicillin. NB: surgical debridement of devitalised tissue is essential. Hyperbaric oxygen may be useful if available. 2. Metronidazole.
Cl. difficile	Antibiotic-associated colitis	1. Oral vancomycin. 2. Metronidazole. NB: well absorbed from the gut so that amount of drug passing into large intestine may be relatively small. Stop other antibiotics if possible.
Bacteroides: *B. fragilis*	Wound sepsis Abscesses and other pyogenic lesions	1. Metronidazole. 2. Clindamycin is also active against anaerobes but is usually avoided because of its potential toxicity
Other bacteroides spp	Wound sepsis Abscesses and other pyogenic lesions	1. Metronidazole. Most species other than *B. fragilis* are sensitive to penicillin.
Anaerobic streptococci	Wound sepsis Abscesses and other pyogenic lesions	1. Penicillin 2. Metronidazole.

Table 3.3 Susceptibility of other micro-organisms to antibacterial drugs

Organism	Antibiotic treatment 1. 1st choice 2. Alternative(s)
1. Bacteria: Spirochaetes: *Leptospira*	Benzyl penicillin (may clear leptospiraemia but probably does not influence liver or renal damage)
Treponema pallidum	1. Benzyl penicillin 2. Erythromycin
Borrelia vincenti	1. Penicillin 2. Metronidazole
Mycobacteria: *M. tuberculosis*	Rifampicin Streptomycin (also agents mainly active against mycobacteria including isoniazid, pyrazinamide, etc.)
M. leprae	Rifampicin Dapsone (a sulphone)
2. Mycoplasma: *Mycoplasma pneumoniae*	Tetracycline Erythromycin
3. Rickettsia: *Coxiella burneti*, rickettsia causing typhus, and other rickettsial disease	1. Tetracycline 2. Chloramphenicol

4. Chlamydia:
Chlamydia psittaci
Chlamydia trachomatis
  a. genital tract infections
  b. neonatal ophthalmia
	Tetracycline
	1. Tetracycline
	2. Erythromycin
	Tetracycline or rifampicin eye ointment (also examine and treat parents)

5. Protozoa: *Pneumocystis carini* *Toxoplasma gondi*	Co-trimoxazole (high doses) Pyrimethamine Spiramycin (preferred for treating infections during pregnancy).

4

Bacterial resistance to antibiotics

Widespread emergence of bacterial resistance may threaten the usefulness of antibiotics because organisms can exploit conditions of sustained selective pressure imposed by extensive antibiotic use. This has been recognised since the early days of antimicrobial therapy—introduction of sulphonamides for treatment of gonorrhoea was soon followed by the emergence of sulphonamide-resistant gonococci. Widespread prophylactic administration of penicillin for prevention of pneumonia in New Guinea has induced penicillin resistance in *Streptococcus pneumoniae*.

MECHANISMS OF BACTERIAL RESISTANCE

1. Intrinsic resistance
Some bacteria are always resistant to particular antibiotics as outlined below; however these mechanisms may also be responsible for *acquired* resistance resulting from genetic changes in bacteria (usually as a consequence of exposure to antibiotics).

    a. The *target site* of antibiotic action is *insusceptible* to an antibiotic e.g. dihydrofolate reductase of neisseria species is invariably relatively insensitive to trimethoprim but in other species such as *E. coli* it is usually sensitive.

    b. The bacterial cell is *impermeable* to an antibiotic, denying entry to the site of antibacterial action. Resistance to tetracycline is mediated in this way. Pseudomonas produces a number of antibiotic-inactivating enzymes, but it is also impermeable to most antibiotics except aminoglycosides, polymixins and antipseudomonal beta-lactams (penicillins and cephalosporins active against pseudomonas). Resistance of Gram-negative aerobic bacilli to erythromycin, clindamycin and fusidic acid is due to failure to penetrate the cell wall.

2. Antibiotic-inactivating enzymes

a. Beta-lactamases

Some organisms produce enzymes capable of inactivating penicillins: 80–90% of hospital staphylococci produce penicillinase although the incidence of resistance in community strains is generally somewhat lower. Over one-third of Gram-negative aerobic bacilli isolated from urinary tract infections produce enzymes capable of inactivating penicillins such as ampicillin, amoxycillin, ticarcillin or mezlocillin. A few Gram-negative bacilli also produce enzymes able to destroy cephalosporins, though newer cephalosporins are very resistant to enzyme inactivation. *Bacteroides fragilis* produces beta-lactamases which destroy penicillin, ampicillin and most cephalosporins except cefoxitin and cefotaxime which are relatively resistant to inactivation. A minority of strains of *Haemophilus influenzae* and *Neisseria gonorrhoeae* also produce beta-lactamase and their emergence in the last decade is a disturbing phenomenon. These organisms have probably acquired resistance determinants from other organisms such as *E. coli* as a result of transfer of genetic material during bacterial conjugation (see p. 16).

b. Aminoglycoside-inactivating enzymes

At least 20 such enzymes are recognised. These enzymes are adenylases, acetylases, and phosphotransferases which may modify the structure of the drug so that it cannot penetrate into the bacterial cell and is unable to reach its target site, the ribosome. Amikacin is susceptible to relatively few of these. Although gentamicin is destroyed by a wider range of enzymes than other aminoglycosides, the overall incidence of gentamicin resistance in hospital Gram-negative bacilli in the United Kingdom is no greater than 4%.

c. Chloramphenicol acetylases

These chloramphenicol-inactivating enzymes have been identified in staphylococci and Gram-negative bacilli. The ability of *Salmonella typhi* and *Haemophilus influenzae* to produce chloramphenicol acetylases is a worrying development of recent years.

THE EMERGENCE OF ANTIBIOTIC RESISTANCE IN BACTERIAL POPULATIONS

1. Therapeutic selection

Intensive use of a drug favours the spread (in hospitals or even in the community) of a minority of strains possessing some degree of natural resistance. Resistant mutants may arise spontaneously and their growth is favoured by the presence of an antibiotic to which they are resistant, because competition due to antibiotic-sensitive bacteria is reduced. Penicillinase-producing strains accounted for less than 1% of *Staphylococcus aureus* isolates before the introduction of penicillin but their incidence has risen progressively and they now comprise 80 to 90% of hospital isolates.

Adaptation by genetic mutation also occurs: development of resistance is usually gradual, taking place by small, step-wise reductions in antibiotic susceptibility. Resistance to erythromycin, clindamycin and fusidic acid may emerge in only a few days and is more likely if bacteria are exposed to subtherapeutic levels of antibiotic. Resistance to streptomycin however may occur very quickly by single step mutation. Combination therapy may be used to suppress resistant mutants, as for example in triple antituberculous therapy using isoniazid, ethambutol and rifampicin or streptomycin, since strains of *M. tuberculosis* resistant to all three, or even two of these agents are rare.

2. Transmissible resistance

Genes determining antibiotic resistance may be transferred from a resistant cell to a sensitive one by transduction or conjugation.

Transduction

Transduction is the transfer of genetic material, usually extrachromosomal DNA, by bacteriophages (viruses which infect bacteria). The ability of staphylococci to produce penicillinase is transmitted in this way.

Conjugation

Gram-negative bacilli may carry resistance-determining plasmids which are extrachromosomal strands of DNA, often responsible for multiple antibiotic resistance. If organisms with antibiotic resistance plasmids also possess a gene conferring the ability to conjugate, they may donate resistance to previously sensitive bacteria. This is known as R-factor mediated resistance. R-factors commonly determine the ability of the cell to produce antibiotic-inactivating enzymes. Conjugation usually takes place between bacteria in the gastro-intestinal tract. Plasmids may be transferred between species and in this way enteric pathogens such as *Salmonella typhi* may acquire resistance from commensal flora. R-factors may be lost spontaneously if antibiotics are withdrawn, since they confer no advantage in the absence of selective pressure. Poor control-of-infection measures allowing bacteria to spread in hospital wards where antibiotics are being used intensively promote the emergence of antibiotic resistance. Antibiotics should be prescribed judiciously and every effort made to prevent the transfer of organisms from patient to patient.

5

Strategies in the management of infection

1. EMPIRICAL ANTIBIOTIC THERAPY

Some infections such as diphtheria or gas gangrene may be diagnosed or suspected on clinical grounds and empirical antibiotic therapy should be started as soon as appropriate specimens have been collected for bacteriological examination. Laboratory confirmation may take at least 24 hours so it is important not to delay treatment.

Patients presenting with life-threatening infections require prompt antibiotic therapy and consideration must be given to likely pathogens and their possible origin. For example a patient who becomes hypotensive and febrile after urological surgery is likely to have Gram-negative septicaemia caused by urinary tract pathogens such as *E. coli*. An aminoglycoside (e.g. gentamicin) or one of the newer cephalosporins, such as cefuroxime, are likely to be active against these organisms and are useful drugs for initial 'best-guess' therapy in such patients. Other infections such as pyogenic meningitis, where a limited number of bacteria are usually implicated, can also be treated empirically choosing an agent or agents which will 'cover' likely pathogens. Empirical antibotic therapy for trivial infections, which may be viral in origin, must be avoided.

2. INTERPRETATION OF BACTERIOLOGICAL REPORTS

Clinical diagnostic laboratories usually perform disc sensitivity tests on pathogens isolated from clinical specimens. Such tests offer a quick and usually reliable means of determining whether the infection is likely to respond to recommended doses of antibiotics.

The laboratory may sometimes issue reports which include antibiotic sensitivities of organisms whose significance is uncertain. It is very important that the relevance of isolates is evaluated clinically—discussion between clinician and microbiologist is often helpful, particularly in assessing the possible significance of bacteria from potentially contaminated specimens such as sputa and wound swabs. Antibiotic therapy is usually indicated only if there is clinical evidence of infection. Whenever possible, narrow-spectrum agents should be chosen in preference to broad-spectrum antibiotics.

3. THE PHARMACOLOGY OF ANTIBIOTICS

Factors other than in vitro activity of an antibiotic determine its performance in treatment. It must be given in adequate dosage, by an appropriate route, and must penetrate adequately to the site of infection.

Laboratory results are designed to provide the best guidance for therapy but may at times require skill and experience in interpretation. The choice of antibiotic should always be governed by consideration of clinical and bacteriological aspects of the individual as well as pharmacokinetic properties of a proposed antibiotic.

4. INFECTIONS WHERE ANTIBIOTICS ALONE MAY FAIL TO ERADICATE A PATHOGEN

a. Abscesses and infections in inaccessible sites, such as advanced osteomyelitis, usually require surgical drainage because antibiotics penetrate poorly into collections of pus or devitalised tissue.

b. Obstructive lesions, for example of the urinary or respiratory tracts, may cause failure of antibiotic therapy, because persistent infection behind an obstruction can be difficult to eradicate with antibiotics alone.

c. Infections involving synthetic material in the body rarely respond to antibiotics alone. For example, septicaemia originating from an infected intravenous cannula must be treated by removal of the cannula, and a suitable antibiotic given if necessary. Infected hip prostheses and CSF valves for drainage of hydrocephalus must usually be removed if they become infected. Urinary infections in patients with indwelling urethral catheters are very difficult to eradicate with antibiotics (but usually require no antibiotic treatment in the absence of symptoms).

d. Defective host immunity may lead to failure of antibiotic treatment. For example severely neutropenic patients with septicaemia may fail to respond to antibiotics shown by the laboratory to be active against pathogens isolated. Synergistic combinations of bactericidal agents are often required in such patients because, in the absence of effective phagocytosis, the outcome depends entirely on the ability of antibiotics to destroy bacteria.

5. THE EFFECTS OF INTENSIVE INDISCRIMINATE ANTIBIOTIC USE ON BACTERIAL RESISTANCE

Sustained selective pressure imposed by the indiscriminate use of antimicrobials promotes the emergence of antibiotic-resistant bacteria. It is important to preserve the value of antibiotics by careful prescribing which is also important if unnecessary toxicity and cost are to be avoided. One of the greatest areas of over-zealous use of antimicrobials is in prophylaxis, and so it is essential to limit prophylactic use of antibiotics to situations where there is good evidence of their value.

6. DURATION OF TREATMENT

In general, the length of course depends on the response of the individual to treatment and type of infection. Long courses should be avoided except for certain serious infections such as endocarditis, osteomyelitis and tuberculosis. Short courses of antibiotics in high doses are usually best for the treatment of acute infections.

6

Antibiotics in combination

The indications for prescribing two antibacterial drugs together are limited. They include:

1. Initial therapy of severe undiagnosed infection before a pathogen has been identified, in order to 'cover' a wide range of possible bacteria.
2. Treatment of mixed infections.
3. To prevent the development of resistance to certain antibiotics. For example, isoniazid, ethambutol and rifampicin are used together in the treatment of tuberculosis to suppress emergence of drug-resistant mutants.
4. To achieve synergy (or greater antimicrobial activity than the sum of the single agents). For example, the most active treatment of a serious Gram-negative chest infection might be achieved by a combination of an aminoglycoside and broad-spectrum penicillin such as mezlocillin, two antibiotics showing synergy against many Gram-negative bacilli in vitro.

Principles of antibiotic interaction were formulated by Jawetz in 1952 who proposed the following:

1. Two bacteristatic drugs* react to produce an additive effect.
2. A bacteristatic and bactericidal†, drug together may be antagonistic.

---

* Bacteristatic antibiotics inhibit the growth of bacteria but do not actively kill them (this is usually accomplished by polymorphs). Bacteristatic antibiotics include tetracycline and chloramphenicol.
† Bactericidal antibiotics kill bacteria and should always be used when the host inflammatory response is inefficient and unable to eradicate organisms only inhibited by bacteristatic antibiotics. For example bactericidal antibiotics are needed in treatment of endocarditis (infection which involves avascular tissue where the host immune response and antibiotic penetration are poor) and in neutropenic patients. In simple infections there is probably little advantage in using a bactericidal agent, since polymorphs effectively destroy bacteria whose growth has been arrested by bacteristatic antibiotics. Bactericidal antibiotics include the penicillins, cephalosporins and aminoglycosides.

3. Two bactericidal drugs together may be synergistic.

These observations have been confirmed only to some extent by clinical data, (e.g. tetracycline has been shown to antagonise penicillin in the treatment of pneumococcal meningitis), but their universal validity remains uncertain. Probably much depends on the individual susceptibility of particular organisms and relative concentrations of drugs, which vary according to their penetration to the site of infection. Synergy between penicillin and gentamicin against streptococci causing endocarditis has been demonstrated in animal experiments as well as in vitro and is exploited in the treatment of human endocarditis. In this infection, penicillin-sensitive streptococci may be killed more rapidly by a combination of penicillin and gentamicin than by penicillin alone, and so both drugs are often used together at least initially (gentamicin is usually stopped once the infection is brought under control).

Disadvantages of antibiotic combinations

The unwanted effects of combined therapy—suppression of normal flora, increased risk of secondary infection caused by resistant organisms, obscured diagnosis, adverse drug reactions and greater cost should always be balanced against possible advantages when using antibiotic combinations. It is important that broad-spectrum antibiotic thereapy should not induce a false sense of security or promote a tendency to dismiss the need for early and accurate bacteriological diagnosis of infection.

7

Properties and use of antimicrobial agents

THE PENICILLINS

Naturally-occurring penicillin obtained from fermentation products of *Penicillium* mould is still the drug of first choice for treatment of infection caused by non-penicillinase-producing staphylococci, streptococci, pneumococci, clostridia, actinomyces and neisseria. It is bactericidal in action and has a very wide margin of safety, so that large doses may be given. Semi-synthetic penicillins such as phenoxymethyl penicillin (penicillin V) derived from the penicillin nucleus are acid-stable and may be taken orally. Cloxacillin and flucloxacillin are stable to staphylococcal beta-lactamases because their side chains protect the beta-lactam ring from enzyme inactivation. Other modifications of the penicillin molecule have produced broad-spectrum acid-stable drugs such as ampicillin and penicillins active against pseudomonas, including carbenicillin, ticarcillin, mezlocillin, azlocillin and piperacillin.

BENZYLPENICILLIN (Penicillin G)

Activity
Active against non-penicillinase-producing staphylococci; streptococci, except *Streptococcus faecalis*, (which is relatively insensitive); pneumococci are almost always highly sensitive, but a few strains with reduced sensitivity have been reported in the UK. (Penicillin-resistant pneumococci have caused serious epidemic infection in South Africa and New Guinea); meningococci; gonococci, except a minority of strains which produce penicillinase; *Actinomyces israeli*; clostridia; spirochaetes (leptospira, *Treponema pallidum*).

Principal uses
Infections caused by organisms listed above including pneumococcal pneumonia, severe streptococcal upper respiratory tract infections,

streptococcal skin infections, streptococcal endocarditis, meningo-coccal and pneumococcal meningitis.

Administration

Adults
IM: 600 mg 6 hourly
IV: up to 24 g daily in divided doses at 4 to 6 hour intervals.

Children (up to 12 years)
IM: 15–20 mg/kg daily.
IV: 15–20 mg/kg 6 hourly for serious sepsis.

Neonates
IM or IV: 15–20 mg/kg 12 hourly.

Benzylpenicillin has a relatively short half-life—its activity may be prolonged by giving probenicid 500 mg–1 g by mouth with each dose to block tubular excretion (or doses may be given 4 hourly in the treatment of severe infection).

Diffusion into CSF is poor, but improved in the presence of meningeal inflammation. Penetration into glandular secretions is limited (for example, penicillin cannot be relied upon to eradicate meningococci from the nasopharynx in asymptomatic carriers, so other agents must be used in prophylaxis of contacts of meningococcal infection; see p. 85).

Principal side effects
Allergy (usually urticarial rashes occurs in between 1 and 7% of patients treated); anaphylaxis occurs rarely. High doses in patients with renal impairment may be associated with hyperkalaemia or neurotoxicity (convulsions etc).

PHENOXYMETHYL PENICILLIN (Penicillin V)

An acid-resistant penicillin; however absorption from the gastro-intestinal tract is incomplete (only about 25%) and inadequate to treat serious infections, where parenteral penicillin is required. Absorption is greater in the fasting state.

Activity
Similar to benzylpenicillin, but is less active than benzylpenicillin against streptococci and considerably less active against neisseria species.

Principal uses
Useful when an oral penicillin is indicated for treatment of relatively mild infections (more severe streptococcal infections require parenteral penicillin).
Streptococcal pharyngitis, sinusitis, otitis media.
Prophylaxis of streptococcal pharyngitis in patients who have had rheumatic fever (see p. 84).
Streptococcal skin infections (NB, penicillin may fail to eradicate sensitive streptococci if penicillinase-producing staphylococci are also present).

Administration

Adults
Oral: 250–500 mg 6 hourly at least 30 minutes before food.

Children
Oral: 62.5–250 mg 6 hourly.

Principal side effects
Hypersensitivity.
Severe reactions are much rarer than with parenteral penicillins.

PROCAINE PENICILLIN

Procaine penicillin is a compound of penicillin and procaine in crystalline suspension, absorbed slowly following intramuscular injection; peak levels are achieved after 4 hours and therapeutic blood levels may persist for 18 to 24 hours.

Activity
As for benzylpenicillin.

Principal uses
Syphilis, gonorrhoea, prophylaxis of gas gangrene. Procaine penicillin may be useful where it is desirable to avoid frequent injections.

Administration
Do not give procaine penicillin intravenously because pulmonary capillaries may become blocked by crystals.
By IM injection   : 300 mg 12–24 hourly.
Syphilis   : 1.2 g daily for 10–21 days.
Gonorrhoea:
  Males   : 2.4 g ⎫
  Females   : 4.8 g ⎭ single dose treatment.

Principal side effects
Hypersensitivity.

Triplopen
This is a mixture of benethamine, benzyl and procaine penicillins which is given by intramuscular injection. Antibacterial activity is induced rapidly by benzylpenicillin and is sustained by the longer-acting components. Single doses are required every 2 or 3 days for treatment of penicillin-sensitive infections. Gonorrhoea may be treated by single injection (2 vials) with probenicid by mouth.

CLOXACILLIN AND FLUCLOXACILLIN

These are isoxazolyl penicillins which are acid-stable and resistant to inactivation by staphylococcal beta-lactamase. They may be given by mouth or parenterally.

Cloxacillin is less efficiently absorbed from the gastro-intestinal tract than flucloxacillin which is therefore preferable for oral therapy. The antibacterial properties of both drugs are similar, although there is some evidence that cloxacillin is more stable to beta-lactamase.

Activity
Active against staphylococci. A minority of isolates of *S. aureus* in the UK are resistant (<3%). Susceptibility of coagulase-negative staphylococci is less predictable. For technical reasons, methicillin is used in laboratory sensitivity tests and resistant strains may be referred to as methicillin-resistant staphylococci. Also active against pyogenic streptococci (but less active than penicillin).

Principal uses
Staphylococcal infections, except those caused by penicillin-sensitive strains (since penicillin is much more active against these organisms). In serious staphylococcal infection involving deep sites eg osteomyelitis or endocarditis, a second drug such as fusidic acid or clindamycin should be used as an adjunct to flucloxacillin, whose high degree of protein-binding may limit its effectiveness in some infections.

Administration Flucloxacillin

Adults
Oral/IV: 250 mg–1 g 6 hourly
IM: 250 mg 6 hourly

Children
Oral/IM/IV: $\frac{1}{4}$ to $\frac{1}{2}$ adult dose

Principal side effects
Hypersensitivity.

AMPICILLIN

A broad spectrum semi-synthetic acid-stable penicillin. Only about one-third of an oral dose is absorbed from the gastro-intestinal tract to yield active drug in the circulation, so it is important to give full therapeutic doses, according to the site of infection (for example, low doses are usually effective in treatment of sensitive urinary infections since large concentrations of antibiotics are excreted into urine; higher doses are needed for chest infection, to ensure therapeutic levels in respiratory secretions, since levels equivalent to between ⅕ and ¹⁄₂₀ of the serum level are achieved in sputum).

Activity
Broad-spectrum activity, including Gram-positive and Gram-negative bacteria. Approximately one-third of Gram-negative aerobic bacilli are resistant even outside hospitals. Ampicillin is destroyed by beta-lactamases of Gram-negative bacilli and staphylococci.

Ampicillin is slightly less active than benzylpenicillin against *Streptococcus pyogenes* and *Streptococcus pneumoniae*. It is active against *Streptococcus faecalis* and most strains of *Haemophilus influenzae*.

Use of ampicillin may suppress normal oral flora leading to colonisation by klebsiellae and other ampicillin-resistant coliforms.

Principal uses
Bronchitis, bacterial pneumonia. Urinary tract infections caused by sensitive bacteria. Upper respiratory tract infections; sinusitis, otitis media. Until recently ampicillin was the drug of choice for invasive *H. influenzae* infections caused by capsulated type b strains in children: however ampicillin resistance in these organisms is now found in about 10% of strains in the UK, so that most paediatricians prefer chloramphenicol for serious infections when sensitivities are unknown.

Administration

Adults
Oral/IV: 250 mg–1 g 6 hourly. Give oral doses at least 30 minutes before food.
IM: 250 mg–500 mg 4–6 hourly.

Children
Oral/IM/IV: Up to half adult dose 6 hourly. Higher doses required for treatment of meningitis.

Principal side effects

Hypersensitivity (usually maculo-papular rashes). NB: almost 100% of patients with infectious mononucleosis, lymphatic leukaemia or lymphoma develop a rash when given ampicillin. Ampicillin should not be given for undiagnosed throat infections. An ampicillin rash is not an absolute contraindication to subsequent treatment with penicillin. Gastro-intestinal side effects, usually diarrhoea.

Fixed-ratio combination penicillins

Combinations of ampicillin and cloxacillin or flucloxacillin are available to simplify medication for patients for whom both drugs are indicated. Before prescribing these preparations, careful consideration must be given to their value for individual cases, taking into account likely pathogen(s), site of infection and dose required for effective treatment. They should not be used as 'umbrella' therapy for undiagnosed infection unless there is good reason to do so and the doses are appropriate.

AMOXYCILLIN

Very closely related to ampicillin in molecular structure with a similar antibacterial spectrum though there is some experimental evidence of superior bactericidal activity; absorbed twice as efficiently when given by mouth. It is however more expensive than ampicillin, so it may often seem reasonable to prescribe high doses of ampicillin; amoxycillin could be chosen for more serious infections when oral therapy is preferred. It may have advantages in the management of chest infections because sputum penetration of amoxycillin has been shown to be superior to that of ampicillin (at least into mucoid sputum; both drugs penetrate purulent sputum to a similar degree). Diarrhoea occurs less frequently with amoxycillin than with ampicillin.

Absorption is not influenced by food and it may be given 8 hourly.

Principal uses
As for ampicillin. Also used in oral prophylaxis of endocarditis (see p. 84).

Administration

Adults
Oral: 250 mg–750 mg 8 hourly.
2-dose treatment of urinary tract infection: 1 single 3 g dose repeated after 12 hours.

Children
Oral: Half adult dose.
An injectable preparation is available but is expensive; ampicillin should usually be chosen for parenteral therapy.

AUGMENTIN

A combination of potassium clavulanate (125 mg) and amoxycillin (250 mg).

Clavulanate has a molecular structure similar to penicillin but has little useful antibacterial activity. It is a powerful inhibitor of beta-lactamases of both Gram-positive and Gram-negative bacteria and protects amoxycillin from inactivation by these enzymes, (which are produced by most staphylococci and over one-third of coliform bacilli).

Activity
The broad-spectrum activity of amoxycillin is extended by clavulanate to include penicillinase-producing staphylococci, a wide range of Gram-negative aerobic bacilli and anaerobes (including *B. fragilis*), as well as other organisms such as streptococci which are sensitive to amoxycillin alone.

Principal uses
Urinary tract infections (if other cheaper drugs are unsuitable or if urine culture and sensitivity are not feasible). Upper and lower respiratory tract infections (although most respiratory pathogens are sensitive to ampicillin or amoxycillin alone).

NB: Augmentin is more expensive than ampicillin or amoxycillin which should be preferred for treatment of sensitive infections.

Administration

Adults
Oral: 1–2 tablets 8 hourly.

Principal side effects
Hypersensitivity.
Gastro-intestinal symptoms.

AMPICILLIN ESTERS

Talampicillin
Pivampicillin
Bacampicillin

These are pro-drugs, hydrolysed by esterases in the gut mucosa following ingestion to yield ampicillin, producing serum levels two or three times greater than those produced by equimolar doses of oral ampicillin. They were developed to overcome the problems of incomplete absorption of ampicillin. They are expensive and probably have little or no advantage over adequate doses of ampicillin (except possibly a lower incidence of diarrhoea).

ANTI-PSEUDOMONAL PENICILLINS

CARBENICILLIN

The first of the broad-spectrum acid-labile penicillins with anti-pseudomonal activity. It has been superseded by more active agents (ticarcillin, mezlocillin, azocillin, piperacillin). All are very expensive.

Activity
Many Gram-negative bacilli, including pseudomonas, and streptococci, including enterococci. Inactivated by staphylococcal beta-lactamase, therefore inactive against most staphylococci. Also hydrolysed by many Gram-negative beta-lactamases. Some activity against anaerobes.

Principal uses
Now superseded by more active agents.

Principal side effects
Penicillin hypersensitivity.
Sodium overload in high doses.

Carfecillin
An ester of carbenicillin hydrolysed by gut esterases to yield car-

benicillin in the blood after oral administration. Serum levels are not adequate for the treatment of systemic infections but bactericidal levels are achieved in urine.

Activity
As for carbenicillin.

Principal uses
Infections of the lower urinary tract caused by sensitive strains of pseudomonas or other multi-resistant organisms, when oral medication is required and other drugs are not suitable.

Administration
Oral: 500 mg–1 g 8 hourly (before food).

TICARCILLIN

An analogue of carbenicillin, though about twice as active. Whilst it is more active against staphylococci than its competitor mezlocillin, it has limited activity against many klebsiella strains. It is susceptible to beta-lactamase inactivation, although the importance of instability to enzymes of all antibiotics in this group depends on a number of factors, notably the size of the bacterial challenge and the speed of enzyme hydrolysis.

Principal uses
As for mezlocillin (see below)

Administration

Adults
IV: 5 g 6–8 hourly.

Children
IV: 50–100 mg/kg 6 hourly.

Principal side effects
Hypersensitivity.
Sodium overload.

UREIDOPENICILLINS

These are anti-pseudomonal penicillins derived from ampicillin.

MEZLOCILLIN

A ureidopenicillin with greater activity than carbenicillin against a wider range of coliforms, including some klebsiellae. It is also more active against pseudomonas and bacteroides, but is inactivated by beta-lactamases of staphylococci and some Gram-negative bacilli.

Principal uses
Broad-spectrum anti-pseudomonal penicillins are probably most effective when used in combination with an aminoglycoside—these two agents are synergistic against many coliforms and pseudomonas, but should not be mixed together before infusion since the aminoglycoside is inactivated. Indications for such a combination include:
1. Empirical treatment of suspected infection in certain compromised hosts, e.g. febrile neutropenic patients.
2. Gram-negative pneumonia caused by susceptible organisms (a rare but serious infection). An aminoglycoside alone may only just achieve therapeutic levels in respiratory secretions and so synergy between the combination may be valuable.
3. Other rare but difficult Gram-negative infections, e.g. endocarditis, meningitis, deep-seated Gram-negative sepsis.

Administration

Adults
Life-threatening infection IV: 5 g 8 hourly.
Non life-threatening infection IM/IV: 2 g 8 hourly.

Children
See data sheet.

Principal side effects
Penicillin hypersensitivity.
Sodium overload less likely than with carbenicillin or ticarcillin.

AZLOCILLIN

A related compound whose activity is greatest against pseudomonas, although it is less active against other Gram-negative bacilli. It should be reserved for the treatment of serious pseudomonas infections sensitive to azlocillin.

Administration
As for mezlocillin.

Principal side effects
As for mezlocillin.

PIPERACILLIN

A ureidopenicillin-like agent with activity against a wide range of Gram-negative organisms, especially pseudomonas. Also active against haemophilus and anaerobes, but rather less activity than other ureidopenicillins against Gram-positive cocci. Like the other drugs in this group, it may be inactivated by beta-lactamases.

Principal uses
As for mezlocillin.

Administration

Adults
IV: 2–4 g, 6–8 hourly according to severity of infection.
The intramuscular route may be used for smaller doses.

Principal side effects
As for mezlocillin.

MECILLINAM AND PIVMECILLINAM

Mecillinam is an amidino-penicillin, also available as the ester pivmecillinam which is taken orally and hydrolysed by gut esterases to yield mecillinam in the circulation.

Activity
Very active against a wide range of Gram-negative bacilli (excluding pseudomonas) but inactive against most Gram-positive organisms.

Principal uses
Urinary tract infections caused by bacteria resistant to other oral antibiotics. Enteric fever; other invasive salmonella infections.

Administration
Pivmecillinam:

Adults
Oral: 200 mg 8 hourly to 600 mg 6 hourly. Higher doses for salmonellosis.

Children
Oral: 30–60 mg/kg per day in divided doses.
Mecillinam:

Adults
IM/IV: 5–15 mg/kg 6 hourly.

Children
IM/IV: 5–15 mg/kg 6 hourly.
(See data sheet)

Principal side effects
Penicillin hypersensitivity.

THE CEPHALOSPORINS

These are drugs with broad-spectrum bactericidal activity, each differing to some extent in antimicrobial and pharmacokinetic behaviour from other members of the group. Pharmaceutical chemists are adept at modifying the molecular structure of these compounds to produce semisynthetic agents with improved antimicrobial and pharmacokinetic properties. There are relatively few specific indications for their use; they should be regarded as useful 'reserve' antibiotics for situations such as the following:
1. In the treatment of sensitive infections in penicillin-allergic patients. If there is a clear history of severe reactions to penicillin they are best avoided, but cross-allergenicity occurs in only about 8 to 10% of patients hypersensitive to penicillin.
2. For treating infections caused by bacteria resistant to other antibiotics when shown to be sensitive by in vitro tests. The newer cephalospsorins e.g. cefuroxime, cefoxitin and cefotaxime, are very resistant to inactivation by Gram-negative beta-lactamases produced by coliform organisms.
3. As empirical therapy for treating some undiagnosed infections requiring immediate treatment, especially in patients with renal impairment, when it may be difficult to decide on initial aminoglycoside dosage.
4. Short-term per-operative prophylaxis of certain surgical procedures where broad-spectrum cover is indicated (see notes on prophylaxis on p. 87).
  Cephaloridine and cephalothin are now obsolete; they are much more readily destroyed by Gram-negative beta-lactamases than their successors and have been associated with nephrotoxicity, which does

not appear to be a problem with newer cephalosporins. It is important to specify the cephalosporin being used when requesting bacteriological investigation for a patient being treated with one of these antibiotics; sensitivity tests to only a few are undertaken routinely, but individual drugs may be tested against clinical isolates if indicated.

CEPHALOSPORINS FOR ORAL ADMINISTRATION

CEPHALEXIN

An oral cephalosporin which is well absorbed but has a relatively short half-life.

Activity
Broad-spectrum activity including many Gram-negative bacilli, staphylococci and streptococci (excluding *Streptococcus faecalis*) though its activity is generally inferior to that of many parenteral cephalosporins. Limited activity against *H. influenzae*.

Principal uses
Mainly in treatment of urinary tract infections where other agents are unsuitable, e.g. in pregnancy, where a pathogen is resistant to ampicillin and other agents are preferably avoided; or other sensitive infections in penicillin-allergic patients.

Administration

Adults
Oral: 250–500 mg 6 hourly (before food).

Children
Oral: 25–50 mg/kg daily in divided doses.

Principal side effects
Rarely nephrotoxic, risk increases if frusemide is given concurrently.
Hypersensitivity.

CEPHRADINE

Activity
Similar to cephalexin and, like cephalexin, is less active than newer injectable cephalosporins against most bacteria.

Principal uses
As for cephalexin.

Administration
Cephradine may be given by mouth or parenterally.

Adults
Oral: 250–500 mg 6 hourly.
IM/IV: 500 mg–1 g 6 hourly. (Absorption following intramuscular injection is poor and serum levels are lower than those following an equivalent oral dose.)

Children
Oral: 25–50 mg/kg/24 h, as divided doses.
IM/IV: 50–100 mg/kg/24 h, as divided doses.

Principal side effects
Hypersensitivity.

CEFACLOR

Activity
More active against haemophilus and many Gram-negative species than cephalexin or cephradine, but is unstable and loses its activity rather quickly—the implications of this in clinical practice are as yet unknown.

Administration
For oral therapy only.

Adults
Oral: 250–500 mg 8 hourly.

Children
Oral: 20–40 mg/kg/24 h.

Principal side effects
Allergic reactions.

CEPHALOSPORINS FOR PARENTERAL USE

CEFAZOLIN

Activity
As for cephalexin, but has a greater range of activity against Gram-

negative bacilli because of enhanced beta-lactamase stability. High concentrations are achieved in bile.

Principal uses
It may be used in treatment of sensitive infections, where parenteral medication is required, or empirically for community-acquired infections, which are likely to be sensitive (e.g. cholecystitis). It is suitable for prophylaxis of certain biliary and gastric operations and hip replacement, given as *short term* per-operative courses.

Administration

Adults
IM/IV: 500 mg–1 g every 6–12 hours.

Children
IM/IV: 125–250 mg every 8 hours.

Principal side effects
Hypersensitivity occasionally. The newer cephalosporins, unlike their predecessors, are not associated with nephrotoxicity. Nevertheless, dose adjustments should be made in renal failure.

CEFAMANDOLE

Activity
Broad-spectrum activity as for other cephalosporins, with stability to many Gram-negative beta-lactamases but, like cefazolin, somewhat less resistant to enzyme inactivation than other newer agents such as cefuroxime, cefoxitin and cefotaxime.

Principal uses
As for cefazolin.

Administration

Adults
IM/IV: 500 mg–2 g 6 hourly.

Children
IM/IV: 50–100 mg/kg/24 hour in divided doses.

Principal side effects
Hypersensitivity.

CEFUROXIME

Activity and principal uses

1. Treatment of serious Gram-negative infections (other than those caused by pseudomonas) as an alternative to aminoglycosides.

2. May be chosen for treatment of serious undiagnosed chest infections because of its activity against haemophilus, (including beta-lactamase producing strains), pneumococci and Gram-negative aerobic bacilli. Staphylococci are also susceptible but the effectiveness of cefuroxime in staphylococcal pneumonia is uncertain.

3. Treatment of infection caused by penicillinase-producing gonococci.

4. Short term per-operative prophylaxis of certain surgical procedures (see pp. 86–88)

Administration

Adults
IM/IV: 750 mg 8 hourly; up to 1.5 mg 6–8 hourly IV.

Children
IM/IV: 10–30 mg/kg 8 hourly.

Principal side effects
Hypersensitivity.
No evidence of nephrotoxicity, but dosage should be adjusted in moderate or severe renal impairment.

CEFOXITIN

This drug is strictly a cephamycin, originally derived from streptomyces bacteria rather than a cephalosporium mould. Expensive.

Activity

Like cefuroxime it is active against a very wide range of Gram-negative bacilli but is less active against haemophilus; also bactericidal to staphylococci (except methicillin-resistant strains), although it is less active than cefuroxime. Active against streptococci but, in common with other cephalosporins, has little effect on *Strept. faecalis*. It has greater activity against anaerobes (approx. 70–80% anaerobes are susceptible). Stability to beta-lactamases produced by *Bacteroides fragilis* renders these anaerobic bacteria sensitive to cefoxitin.

Principal uses

1. May be used in surgical sepsis because of its wide spectrum of activity against coliforms and anaerobes, although cover is not as

broad as a combination of an aminoglycoside and metronidazole. Higher doses are needed to achieve satisfactory activity against most anaerobes.

2. Undiagnosed bacteraemia where Gram-negative organisms or anaerobes are suspected, if pseudomonas is unlikely.

Administration

Adults
IM/IV: 1–2 g 8 hourly.

Children
IM/IV: 80–160 mg/kg/24 h in divided doses.

Principal side effects
As for cefuroxime. Intramuscular injection is painful; it should preferably be given intravenously.

CEFOTAXIME

Activity
Very active in vitro against Gram-negative bacilli, including some activity against pseudomonas; also active against neisseria, haemophilus, streptococci and staphylococci although activity against Gram-positive organisms is less than cefuroxime. Most anaerobes are relatively sensitive, although high doses are required in treatment.

Principal uses
Serious undiagnosed sepsis, especially in surgical patients where Gram-negative bacilli or anaerobes are likely pathogens. Also treatment of infection caused by sensitive bacteria resistant to other (cheaper) antibiotics.

Its value in pseudomonas infections other than urinary tract infections is uncertain as yet, since adequate tissue levels may be difficult to achieve (high doses are necessary).

Administration

Adults
IM/IV: 1 g 8–12 hourly (maximum 12 g daily IV in 3–4 doses).

Children
IM/IV: 100–150 mg/kg/24 h in 2–4 doses.

Principal side effects
As for cefuroxime.

LATAMOXEF ('MOXALACTAM')

A new cephalosporin-like agent, with very broad-spectrum activity against most Gram-negative bacilli, including some effect on pseudomonas and activity against anaerobes. A notable feature is its relatively good penetration into CSF. Latamoxef should be useful in the treatment of meningitis caused by Gram-negative aerobic bacilli and haemophilus (but not for undiagnosed meningitis because of its relatively poor activity against pneumococci). Also for treatment of infection caused by sensitive bacteria resistant to other (cheaper) antibiotics.

Administration
Adults
IM/IV 500 mg–6 g/24 hours as 2–3 doses.

Principal side effects
Hypersensitivity. Bleeding problems (more likely in elderly or debilitated patients)

CEFSULODIN

Activity
Highly active against *Ps. aeruginosa*, including most strains resistant to gentamicin. Very little activity against other Gram-negative bacilli and Gram-positive organisms.

Principal use
Infection caused by sensitive strains of *Ps. aeruginosa*.

Administration
Adults
IV/IM: 1–4 g daily in 2–4 divided doses.

Children
IV/IM: 20–50 mg/kg/day in divided doses.

CEFTAZIDIME

Activity
A newer extended spectrum parenteral cephalosporin with good

activity against a wide variety of Gram-negative bacilli, including pseudomonas; less active than other cephalosporins against *Staphylococcus aureus*. Bacteroides species may sometimes be only moderately sensitive and even resistant to ceftazidime.

THE AMINOGLYCOSIDES

A valuable group of drugs with bactericidal activity against many Gram-negative bacilli and staphylococci, but inactive against streptococci and anaerobes. Streptomycin is the most active of the group against mycobacteria but unlike newer aminoglycosides has little useful activity against pseudomonas; like kanamycin, it is no longer used in the treatment of acute sepsis. Aminoglycosides must be given parenterally in treatment of systemic infections. Topical use of aminoglycosides also used parenterally is strongly discouraged because of the possibility of selecting resistance, notably to gentamicin, which is active against at least 96% of Gram-negative bacilli in hospitals in the United Kingdom. Aminoglycosides share in varying degrees the tendency to cause renal damage and ototoxicity; the difference between therapeutic and toxic levels is small so that it is often necessary to monitor serum levels in order to control dosage (see p. 89).

New semi-synthetic agents have been developed in attempts to overcome problems of toxicity and to produce agents which are even more resistant to aminoglycoside-inactivating enzymes than gentamicin.

GENTAMICIN

Activity
Active against most Gram-negative bacilli including pseudomonas. Activity against staphylococci is good in vitro although other specifically antistaphylococcal agents are preferred for treatment of staphylococcal infections. Not active against anaerobes or streptococci.

Principal uses
1. Septicaemia, or serious sepsis where Gram-negative bacilli are known or suspected pathogens.
2. Pseudomonas infections.

In certain sites, where bactericidal tissue levels may be difficult to achieve, combination with an antipseudomonal penicillin may be indicated, e.g. Gram-negative pneumonia, Gram-negative endocarditis.

Caution: Do not mix a broad spectrum antipseudomonal penicillin with an aminoglycoside before giving, since the aminoglycoside will be inactivated. This does not occur in vivo except in severe renal impairment.

Administration

Adults
IM/IV: 3–7.5 mg/kg/24 hours in divided doses if renal function is normal. Adjust in renal impairment—see data sheets or nomogram for initial dosage and assay serum levels to determine subsequent dosage (a nomogram is a formula for calculating dosage, based on age, weight, sex and renal function).

Children
Up to 2 weeks of age—IM/IV: 3 mg/kg 12 hourly (Antibiotics are often given twelve-hourly in the first week of life because of immature renal function).
2 weeks to 12 years—2 mg/kg 8 hourly
An account of the laboratory control of antibiotic therapy is given on p. 89. The therapeutic range for peak serum levels is 5–12 mg/l. Trough levels should be less than 2 mg/l. If renal tubular damage occurs failure to excrete gentamicin is often detected before serum creatinine rises. This should be regarded as an indication to adjust dosage or increase the dosage interval.

Principal side effects

Nephrotoxicity—usually a progressive rise in serum creatinine (rather than acute renal failure); it is not usually detectable until at least the fifth day of gentamicin therapy.

Ototoxicity—gentamicin otoxicity is predominantly vestibular, although there may also be hearing loss.

These effects may be reversible on stopping gentamicin as long as high serum and tissue levels are not sustained. Most toxicity is dose-related and therefore avoidable by careful management of dosage. Courses longer than 7 days should be avoided. Previous treatment with aminoglycosides is a risk factor in the development of toxicity. Concurrent use of diuretics such as frusemide is also associated with an increased likelihood of nephrotoxicity.

TOBRAMYCIN

Activity
Tobramycin is about twice as active as gentamicin against pseudomonas, but may be less active against some other Gram-negative species, notably *E. coli*, klebsiella, proteus and serratia.

Administration
As for gentamicin. The therapeutic range of serum levels is similar to that of gentamicin.

Principal side effects
Ototoxicity, nephrotoxicity—tobramycin may be marginally less toxic than gentamicin, but it is still important to manage dosage carefully, particularly in renal impairment and in the elderly.

AMIKACIN

A semi-synthetic derivative of kanamycin with similar pharmacology. Very expensive.

Activity and principal uses
Active against a wider range of Gram-negative bacilli than other aminoglycosides but should be reserved for treatment of infections caused by gentamicin- and tobramycin-resistant organisms.

Administration
Adults and children
IM/IV: 15 mg/kg/day in 2 divided doses. Dose controlled by monitoring serum levels. Therapeutic range 15–30 mg/1. Trough levels should be less than 8 mg/1.

Principal side effects
As for other aminoglycosides, but ototoxicity is predominantly auditory rather than vestibular.

NETILMICIN

A semi-synthetic aminoglycoside derivative.

Activity

Active against a wide range of Gram-negative bacilli including some organisms resistant to gentamicin. It may have less activity than gentamicin against some strains of pseudomonas and serratia.

Administration

Adults
IM/IV: 4–6 mg/kg/24 h in 2 doses.

Principal side effects

Ototoxicity, nephrotoxicity. Evidence suggests that netilmicin is less ototoxic than other aminoglycosides, but the clinical advantage of this is uncertain, since aminoglycoside therapy must be controlled by serum assays in renal impairment and in the elderly.

OTHER AMINOGLYCOSIDES

STREPTOMYCIN

The only indication for streptomycin now is in treatment of tuberculosis in patients unable to tolerate other first-line drugs (see p. 65).

Streptomycin should no longer be used with penicillin in treatment of endocarditis since many strains of *Streptococcus faecalis* are resistant to the synergistic effects of this combination. Gram-negative bacilli may readily acquire resistance to streptomycin.

NEOMYCIN

Neomycin is active against Gram-negative bacilli and most staphylococci. It is too toxic for parenteral use but is sometimes given orally to suppress bowel flora in hepatic failure to prevent encephalopathy or to neutropenic patients as part of gut decontamination programmes. Small amounts may be absorbed from the gut so caution is needed in patients with renal failure.

Administration

1. Oral: 1 g 4 hourly.
2. Topical application, e.g. as cream in combination with chlorhexidine (Naseptin) for treatment of staphylococcal nasal carriage. Also eye preparations for bacterial conjunctivitis and ear drops for otitis externa. NB, long-term topical use may generate resistance.

FRAMYCETIN

Framycetin is neomycin B, identical to neomycin in antibacterial activity.

Framycetin is sometimes given by mouth as part of gut decontamination programmes to reduce endogenous bacteria in neutropenic patients. It may also be applied topically.

SPECTINOMYCIN

An aminocyclitol: a bactericidal antibiotic with a structure similar to the aminoglycosides.

Activity
Gram-negative bacteria including *Neisseria gonorrhoeae*. Inactive against chlamydia or treponemes.

Principal use
Its only indication is for treatment of penicillin-resistant *N. gonorrhoeae* or gonorrhoea in penicillin-allergic patients.

Administration
IM: 2 to 4 g as single dose.

Principal side effects
Very unlikely when given as a single dose.

MACROLIDES AND LINCOSAMIDES

ERYTHROMYCIN

A macrolide antibiotic which is generally bacteristatic against susceptible bacteria at low concentrations but bactericidal at high levels.

Activity
Active against Gram-positive bacteria including staphylococci, streptococci, pneumococci. Also active against haemophilus, *Bordetella pertussis*, campylobacter and *Legionella pneumophila*.

PRINCIPAL USES

May be used in penicillin-hypersensitive patients for treatment of staphylococcal sepsis, streptococcal pharyngitis, sinusitis, otitis media and lower respiratory tract infections.

Also: diphtheria; whooping cough; legionnaires' disease; campylobacter enteritis; mycoplasma and chlamydial infections as an alternative to tetracycline.

Administration

Erythromycin base is acid labile, so must be given as an enteric-coated preparation; even so, absorption may be delayed or incomplete. Alternatively the stearate or estolate may be given—higher serum erythromycin levels are achieved using the estolate—but the drug is potentially hepatotoxic. The ethylsuccinate is available as a suspension for children.

Erythromycin may be given intramuscularly as the ethylsuccinate, but this route is best avoided because it is painful and not suitable for doses exceeding 100 mg. (Erythromycin in this form is relatively insoluble and large volumes of diluent are required to dissolve higher doses). The intramuscular preparation is no longer available in the United Kingdom.

Erythromycin lactobionate or glucoheptonate are used when intravenous infusion is required.

Adults
Oral: 250–500 mg 6 hourly.
IV (erythromycin lactobionate): 300 mg–1.2 g 6 hourly.
NB: High doses are needed in Legionnaires' disease and certain other serious infections, e.g. 1 g 6 hourly.

Children
Oral: 125–250 mg 6 hourly.

Principal side effects

Gastro-intestinal side effects.
The estolate is particularly associated with jaundice especially following prolonged use (>10 days), although other forms of erythromycin may also cause liver damage occasionally. High dosage in patients with renal failure has caused ototoxicity.

CLINDAMYCIN

A 7-chloro derivative of lincomycin which is much more active than the parent compound. Clindamycin has close structural similarity to macrolides such as erythromycin, and shows similar antibacterial activity.

Activity
Active against staphylococci and streptococci (excluding *Strept. faecalis*). Good activity against anaerobes.

Principal uses
A useful drug for deep-seated staphylococcal infection, such as osteomyelitis and staphylococcal pneumonia, or serious mixed infections including synergistic gangrene (often caused by staphylococci or streptococci and anaerobes), because of its good tissue penetration. In serious staphylococcal infection it may be used as an adjunct or alternative to flucloxacillin whose high degree of protein-binding may limit its effectiveness in certain sites. It is effective in treatment of anaerobic infections but other agents, notably metronidazole, are now preferred because of possible clindamycin-associated colitis.

Administration

Adults
Oral: 150–300 mg 6 hourly:
IM/IV: 600 mg–2.7 g in 24 hours as 2–4 doses.

Children
Oral: 75–150 mg 6 hourly.
IM/IV: 15–40 mg/kg/24 h as 3–4 doses.

Principal side effects
Antibiotic-associated colitis—because of this potentially serious complication, clindamycin should be reserved for treatment of severe infections caused by susceptible organisms or when other drugs are ineffective. The risk is greatest in the elderly and in hospitalised patients. The drug should be withdrawn if diarrohea develops. If symptoms are severe and persistent, stools should be examined for *Cl. difficile* and its toxin and, if necessary, treatment for antibiotic-associated colitis instituted (see p. 12)

SODIUM FUSIDATE

Activity
Very active against *Staphylococcus aureus* but no clinically useful activity against other species.

Principal uses

Good bone and tissue penetration, and so useful in osteomyelitis and other deep-seated staphylococcal infections.

Resistance may emerge if it is used alone, therefore most authorities suggest that it should be combined with another antibiotic, e.g. flucloxacillin or penicillin.

Administration

It is advisable to use the oral route if possible, since the drug is well absorbed from the gastro-intestinal tract. Local use encourages the emergence of resistance and should be avoided.

Adults
Oral: 500 mg 8 hourly.
IV: 500 mg infused over 6 hours, at 8 hourly intervals.

Children
Oral: see data sheet.
IV: 20 mg/kg/day infused slowly as 3 divided doses.

Principal side effects

Nausea, vomiting, rashes, jaundice (disturbance of liver function may be more common after IV administration).

POLYMIXINS (including colistin)

Peptide antibiotics, active against a wide range of Gram-negative bacilli, including pseudomonas; these agents have now been superseded by aminoglycosides and broad-spectrum penicillins for treatment of systemic pseudomonas infections. There are few indications for their use today.

Topical preparations of polymixin may be considered in management of superficial infections if pseudomonas is a problem, e.g. otitis externa. Topical antibiotics should usually be avoided, because they promote the emergence of resistance but since polymixin is almost never used for systemic therapy nowadays and resistance to polymixins is not at present a problem, the usual objection is probably not applicable.

Principal side effects (associated with systemic therapy)

Nephrotoxicity.
Neurotoxicity (paraesthesiae, dizziness, muscle weakness).
These effects are usually reversible.

THE SULPHONAMIDES

Broad-spectrum synthetic bacteristatic antimicrobials, with largely similar antibacterial activity but differing in pharmacological behaviour.
  Most practitioners need to be familiar with only a few of these compounds.

Activity

Bacteristatic against Gram-negative bacilli (although at least one-third of isolates are resistant), meningococci, haemophilus. Increasing resistance in many species has followed extensive use of sulphonamides and so their applications have become more limited.

SULPHADIAZINE

Sulphadiazine has been chosen in preference to other sulphonamides when required for treatment of meningococcal meningitis because of its relatively low degree of protein binding, which facilitates diffusion into CSF. Sulphonamides penetrate CSF quite readily. The parenteral form is marketed in the United Kingdom, although sulphadiazine is also available combined with trimethoprim as co-trimazine and as other combined sulphonamide preparations for oral use.

SULPHADIMIDINE AND SULPHAFURAZOLE

These drugs are used in treatment of urinary tract infections caused by susceptible organisms. Sulphadimidine is a general purpose sulphonamide, and has been preferred by some for treatment of meningitis because it is less often associated with crystalluria and renal blockage than sulphadiazine. Its antibacterial activity however tends to be lower than that of sulphadiazine. Sulphafurazole is the most soluble in urine.

Principal uses:

1. Urinary tract infection (caused by susceptible strains).
2. Meningococcal meningitis (sometimes in combination with penicillin, although penicillin alone is usually preferable). NB: about 15% of strains of *N. meningitidis* are sulphonamide-resistant in the UK and so sulphonamides are no longer drugs of choice

either in treatment or prophylaxis, unless isolates are known to be sulphonamide-sensitive.
3. Nocardial infection.

Administration of sulphonamides

Adults
Sulphadimidine (oral, IM or IV) and sulphafurazole (oral) for UTI: 2 g initially then 1 g 6 hourly.
Sulphadiazine: 3 g or 50/mg/kg initially, then 100 mg/kg/day, IM/IV for meningococcal meningitis caused by sensitive strains.

Principal side effects
Rashes, crystalluria, blood dyscrasias, haemolytic anaemia, rarely Stevens-Johnson syndrome, nausea, vomiting. Contra-indicated in pregnancy and infants under 6 weeks because of possible effect on folate metabolism and because sulphonamides may displace bilirubin from serum proteins, resulting in kernicterus in the newborn.

SILVER SULPHADIAZINE

Used prophylactically in severe burns to prevent infection caused by a wide spectrum of bacteria, including pseudomonas. Resistance may emerge during use.

Administration
Local application of cream daily: apply a layer of about 3–5 mm with aseptic precautions.

CO-TRIMOXAZOLE

Sulphamethoxazole and trimethoprim combined in a ratio of 5: 1 intended to give maximum synergy against many bacteria in tissue (this is said to occur when the two components are present in a ratio of 20: 1 although in fact much depends on the strain concerned). A synergistic ratio between both components may not always be achieved because of differences in penetration to particular sites.

Activity
Active against most Gram-negative bacilli (except *Pseudomonas aeruginosa*), staphylococci, streptococci, haemophilus, *N. gonorrhoeae*.

Not reliably active against anaerobes, which are intrinsically insusceptible to trimethoprim.

Principal uses
1. Urinary tract infections, although there are strong arguments now for preferring trimethoprim alone see p. 52.
2. Respiratory tract infections.
3. Sinusitis, otitis media.
   (NB: Trimethoprim alone will possibly replace co-trimoxazole in treatment of respiratory infections also.)
4. Gonorrhoea in penicillin-allergic patients.
5. Invasive salmonella infections.
6. Pneumocystis pneumonia.

Administration

Adults
Oral: 2 tablets (960 mg) 12 hourly (each tablet contains 400 mg sulphamethoxazole and 80 mg trimethoprim).
IM/IV: 960 mg 12 hourly (960 mg contains 800 mg sulphamethoxazole and 160 mg trimethoprim).

Children
Oral: 6–12 years—half adult dose (suspension or tablets)
IV: see data sheet.

Pneumocystis pneumonia
For treatment of pneumocystis pneumonia large doses are needed:

Adults
Oral: 12 tablets daily in 4 divided doses.

Children
Oral: sulphamethoxazole 25 mg/kg + trimethoprim 5 mg/kg, 6 hourly.

In prophylaxis of susceptible individuals with impaired cell-mediated immunity normal therapeutic doses are used.

Principal side effects
Nausea, vomiting, rashes, blood dyscrasias, rarely Stevens-Johnson syndrome. Contra-indicated in pregnancy and infants less than 6 weeks.

TRIMETHOPRIM

Currently recommended for treatment of urinary tract and respiratory infections, but applications may extend to other conditions, since tissue penetration of trimethoprim is generally good, and its activity includes a broad-spectrum of pathogens (see below).

Use of trimethoprim alone means that unnecessary risk of sulphonamide toxicity is avoided. The sulphonamide component in co-trimoxazole is often redundant, since at least one-third of isolates from UTIs are resistant to sulphonamides. Furthermore, a synergistic ratio is frequently not achieved in urine when co-trimoxazole is given, so that in many cases antibacterial activity in urine is only that of trimethoprim.

A potential problem of widespread use of trimethoprim is that resistance may emerge more readily. It is not known whether combination with a sulphonamide delays the evolution of resistance to trimethoprim. Resistance trends must be monitored locally since there is some evidence from UK studies that resistance does emerge, albeit slowly.

Activity
A wide range of Gram-negative bacilli are susceptible. Currently between 10–26% of isolates from UTIs are resistant. Most strains resistant to trimethoprim are also sulphonamide-resistant. Also active against most staphylococci, streptococci and haemophilus. Anaerobes and neisseria are intrinsically resistant to trimethoprim.

Principal uses
Urinary tract infections, respiratory tract infections.

Administration

Adults
Oral: 200 mg 12 hourly.
IV: 150–250 mg (by slow IV) 12 hourly.

Children
Oral: 6–12 years—half adult dose.
IV: 6–9 mg/kg/day as 2 divided doses.

Principal side effects
Skin rashes, nausea, vomiting unusual. Folate deficiency and

depression of haemopoeisis—although human folate metabolism is much less susceptible to antagonism by trimethoprim than bacterial folate synthesis. It is contra-indicated in pregnancy and neonates.

New combinations of sulphonamindes and trimethoprim
Other sulphonamide/trimethoprim combinations are now available in addition to co-trimoxazole. These use sulphonamides whose pharmacological behaviour may make them more appropriate partners for trimethoprim (for example sulphadiazine produces levels in urine twice those of sulphamethoxazole). Their real advantage in clinical practice is still uncertain.

CHLORAMPHENICOL

Activity
A broad-spectrum, predominantly bacteristatic antibiotic, active against a wide range of Gram-negative bacilli (excluding pseudomonas), staphylococci, streptococci, haemophilus and anaerobes. Originally produced from a soil streptomycete, it is now manufactured synthetically.

Principal uses
Chloramphenicol should be prescribed for serious sensitive infections for which there is no alternative therapy:
1. Meningitis caused by coliforms or haemophilus, and in some cases of undiagnosed bacterial meningitis. Chloramphenicol diffuses well into CSF.
2. Other serious infectious caused by capsulated strains of *H. influenzae* such as epiglottitis and pneumonia in young children.
3. Typhoid—chloramphenicol is still the best drug for severe infection, because of its efficient penetration into cells, (typhoid is a predominantly intracellular infection). Milder cases of typhoid should usually be treated with other agents such as co-trimoxazole or mecillinam.
4. Treatment of some patients with brain abscess (particularly if otogenic) where multiple pathogens including anaerobes are likely.
5. Topical use as eye drops for treatment of bacterial conjunctivitis.

Administration
Parenteral administration may be less frequently associated with toxicity than oral therapy. Chloramphenicol is very well absorbed after oral administration, giving levels similar to those following IV injection. The palmitate suspension should be avoided in neonates

because of the possibility of incomplete absorption; it is tasteless and therefore useful for children, who may not tolerate the bitter parent compound.

Adults
Oral: 500 mg 6 hourly before food.
IM/IV: 50–100 mg/kg/day in 4 divided doses

Children
Neonates IV/IM: 25 mg/kg daily at 6 to 12 hourly intervals (12 hourly dosage for premature babies and during the first week of life). Full-term infants over 2 weeks IV/IM: 25–50 mg/kg daily in 4 doses.
6/12 months–5 years IV/IM: 50–100 mg/kg daily in 4 doses.
   NB: absorption following intramuscular injection is slow, peak levels occurring after 2 to 5 hours. This route should be avoided because levels achieved in serum are lower than those following equivalent oral doses.
   Courses should extend for no longer than 10 days.
   Chloramphenicol eye drops—give 2 drops every 3 hours. Eye ointment—1 application every 3 hours.

Principal side effects
1. Irreversible aplastic anaemia; an idiosyncrasy, not dose dependent. The risk is approximately one in 25 000 doses.
2. Reversible, dose-dependent marrow depression, which is relatively common. There is no apparent relationship between this and the rare aplastic anaemia. Blood counts should be monitored regularly during treatment.
3. 'Grey baby syndrome' in neonates is dose related, therefore it is important to monitor serum chloramphenicol levels (the therapeutic range is usually given as 10–50 mg/l although since peak levels need not exceed 30 mg/l for therapeutic effect, it may be wise to maintain levels below 30 mg/l in premature babies to ensure an extra margin of safety). Trough serum levels should not exceed 15 mg/l.
4. Nausea, vomiting, diarrhoea.

TETRACYCLINES

Broad-spectrum bacteristatic antimicrobials, whose value has been reduced of late because of increasing bacterial resistance especially in respiratory pathogens.

There is little difference in their microbiological activity except for minocycline, which is more active against *Staphylococcus aureus* and *N. meningitidis* and shows some enhanced activity against a number of other organisms.

Doxycycline does not exacerbate renal failure, although other tetracyclines should not be used in patients with kidney disease because they may cause deterioration in renal function.

Tetracyclines are chelated by calcium and other metal ions and should therefore not be given with milk, antacids, calcium, iron or magnesium salts which may impair absorption.

TETRACYCLINE

Activity
Active against coliforms, streptococci, pneumococci and staphylococci, although resistance has increased. Approximately one-third of haemolytic streptococci are tetracycline-resistant. Tetracyclines have important activity against mycoplasmas, rickettsia, chlamydia and brucella.

Principal uses
1. Non-specific urethritis and chlamydial infections including psittacosis.
2. Exacerbations of chronic bronchitis (when pathogens are known to be sensitive).
3. Severe acne vulgaris.
4. Brucellosis.
5. Mycoplasma infection.
6. Rickettsial disease (Q fever, typhus etc).
7. Cholera.
8. Prophylaxis of meningococcal infection (minocycline).

Administration

Adults
Oral: 250–500 mg 6 hourly.
IM: 100–200 mg 6 hourly.
IV: 500 mg 12 hourly by slow infusion.

Children
Avoid below the age of 12 because of concentration in teeth and bones.

Principal side effects
Gastro-intestinal disturbances (dose dependent). Candida superin-
fection (because of broad-spectrum suppression of commensal flora).
Exacerbation of renal failure: contra-indicated in patients with renal
disease. Doxycycline may be used in such patients because there is
an alternative route of elimination via the gastro-intestinal tract.
Tooth staining and interference of bone development—do not give
to children under 12 years of age or pregnant women. Tetracyclines
given intravenously in large doses have caused liver damage,
especially in pregnant women.

MINOCYCLINE

Activity and principal uses
Often active against strains of haemophilus, pneumococcus, coliforms and *Staphylococcus aureus* resistant to other tetracyclines. Useful in some patients with exacerbations of chronic bronchits. There
is some evidence that minocycline achieves higher sputum levels
than other tetracyclines. Activity against *N. meningitidis* makes it
useful in prophylaxis of meningococcal infection (see notes on prophylaxis p. 85). It is more expensive than other tetracyclines and
possible advantages must be considered in the light of greater cost.

Administration

Adults
Oral: 200 mg initially then 100 mg every 12 hours.

Children
Avoid.

Principal side effects
As for tetracycline. Vestibular disturbances (vertigo etc.) occur in
10% or more patients; women are apparently more susceptible than
men. It is important to warn patients of this possible side effect particularly when prescribing minocycline for well contacts of meningococcal meningitis or ambulant patients, in whom vertigo may
possibly precipitate an accident.

DOXYCYCLINE

A long-acting tetracycline which does not lead to deterioration in
renal function in patients with renal disease. It may therefore be

useful in the elderly. Also useful in genital tract infections (gonorrhoea or chlamydial infection) since a once daily regime encourages compliance. It is relatively expensive.

Administration

Adults
Oral: 200 mg on first day then 100 mg daily.

OTHER ANTIBACTERIAL DRUGS

VANCOMYCIN

A bactericidal antibiotic active against staphylococci (including methicillin-resistant strains) and streptococci (including *Streptococcus faecalis*) and many clostridia. Vancomycin is not significantly absorbed from the gastro-intestinal tract. It is expensive.

Principal uses
1. A reserve antibiotic for use in some cases of bacterial endocarditis if hypersensitivity to penicillins and cephalosporins precludes use of these drugs.
2. May rarely be needed in treatment of life-threatening infections caused by multi-resistant staphylococci.
3. For *Cl. difficile*-associated colitis, given by mouth.

Administration

Adults
IV: 500 mg 6 hourly over 30 minutes.
   Oral vancomycin for antibiotic-associated colitis where clostridial toxin has been identified: 125–500 mg 6 hourly orally for 5 days.

Children
IV: 44 mg/kg/24 hours in divided doses

Principal side effects (parenteral vancomycin)
Nausea, chills, rashes, fever, eosinophilia. Local irritation at infusion site, thrombophlebitis if the drug extravasates. Ototoxicity (deafness, tinnitus). Nephrotoxicity. Serum levels should be monitored when given systemically (therapeutic range = 5–50 mg/l). If trough levels remain below 5 mg/l toxic effects are minimised; the preparation now available is tolerated better than an earlier formulation.

METRONIDAZOLE

Activity

Active only against anaerobic bacteria and protozoa, although there is some activity against campylobacter spp and *Gardnerella vaginalis* which are not obligate anaerobes. Otherwise it is inactive against micro-aerophilic and aerobic bacteria and aerobic protozoa such as trypanosomes. Resistance may be induced in vitro but is very rare in anaerobes from clinical specimens (it has been found in strains from patients who have received long-term metronidazole). Metronidazole is reduced to an hydroxy-metabolite by anaerobic organisms; its activity is believed to be due to activity of the metabolite.

Principal uses

1. Treatment and prophylaxis of anaerobic sepsis. (Use in surgical prophylaxis is outlined on p. 86–87).
2. Trichomoniasis.
3. Enteric and tissue infections caused by *Entamoeba histolytica*.
4. *Giardia lamblia* enteritis.
5. Vincent's angina (as an alternative to penicillin).
6. Results in treatment of non-specific vaginitis show some promise possibly because of activity against *Gardnerella vaginalis*.

Administration

Metronidazole is well absorbed following oral or rectal administration—these routes should be used whenever possible, since parenteral metronidazole is expensive. A recent survey in the UK has shown that metronidazole accounted for 28% of the total cost of antibiotics in hospitals—this may well reflect prolonged use of intravenous metronidazole in surgical prophylaxis.

Metronidazole administration for anaerobic infection:

Adults

Oral: 400 mg 8 hourly (peak serum levels are achieved after 1 to 4 hours). Or:
Suppository: 1 g 8 hourly for 3 days, then 1 g 12 hourly (peak serum levels are achieved after about 4 hours following rectal administration).
IV: 500 mg in 100 ml over 30 minutes 8 hourly.

Intravenous metronidazole should be reserved for situations requiring high serum levels immediately or for difficult infections, e.g. anaerobic endocarditis where bacteria may be relatively inaccessible and highest tissue levels are required initially to control infection. Oral therapy should be substituted as soon as possible.

Children
Oral/rectal: 7.5 mg/kg 8 hourly.
IV: 7.5 mg/kg 8 hourly.

Metronidazole administration for parasitic infections (adult doses): Trichomoniasis—oral: 200 mg 8 hourly for 7 days or oral: 2 g single dose.
Amoebiasis—oral: 800 mg 8 hourly for 5 days.
Giardiasis—oral: 2 g daily for 3 days.

Large doses are needed for enteric infections because efficient absorption from the gut leaves relatively little active drug in the faeces.

Principal side effects
Nausea, usually related to accumulation of drug; individuals may vary in their pharmacological handling of metronidazole and dose reductions may be needed if upper gastro-intestinal disturbance is a problem. These effects may be minimised by taking metronidazole with food. A disulfiram-like effect (flushing and hypotension) may occur in association with alcohol. Prolonged use in high doses may lead to sensory peripheral neuropathy; CNS effects including vertigo, ataxia and convulsions may follow high doses. Contra-indicated in pregnancy (because of a controversial mutagenic effect).

TINIDAZOLE

A nitroimidazole compound with an antimicrobial spectrum of activity similar to that of metronidazole but with a longer half-life. It is available for oral and intravenous administration.

URINARY ANTIMICROBIALS

NITROFURANTOIN

An oral drug which should be used only in treatment of lower urinary tract infection because serum levels are not adequate (partly because of rapid metabolism) for treatment of systemic infection, including pyelonephritis.

Activity
Active against a wide range of Gram-negative bacilli, excluding

proteus spp and pseudomonas. Also active against Gram-positive urinary pathogens such as staphylococci and *Strept. faecalis*.

Principal use
Lower urinary tract infection.

Administration

Adults
Oral: 100 mg 6 hourly (with food, to suppress the rate of absorption and so to minimise upper gastro-intestinal problems).

Children
Oral: 25–50 mg 6 hourly.

Principal side effects
Nausea, vomiting, rashes, drug fever. Contra-indicated in uraemia (toxic metabolites accumulate and little active drug is excreted into urine). May precipitate haemolysis in patients with G6PD deficiency. Occasionally associated with peripheral neuropathy and acute pneumonitis.

NALIDIXIC ACID

Only for use in lower urinary tract infections because low serum levels are inadequate for treatment of systemic or renal parenchymal infections.

Activity
Active against most Gram-negative bacilli except pseudomonas. Transmissible R-factor mediated resistance in Gram-negatives does not occur, although other mechanisms may be responsible for resistance, which is not uncommon in isolates from patients who have had repeated courses of antibiotics for recurrent urinary infections. Nalidixic acid is inactive against Gram-positive bacteria.

Principal use
Lower urinary tract infections where other cheaper antibiotics are not suitable.

Administration

Adults
Oral: 1 g 6 hourly.

Children
Oral: 250–500 mg 6 hourly, (maximum 50 mg/kg/day)

Principal side effects
Gastro-intestinal irritation. Occasional photosensitivity; raised intra-cranial pressure or convulsions have been reported in infants or patients with CNS abnormalities. Do not use in uraemia because of accumulation of potentially toxic metabolites. Do not give to children under 3 months or to patients with CNS lesions.

CINOXACIN

Similar activity to nalidixic acid, but slightly more active against some Gram-negative organisms.

Administration

Adults
Oral: 500 mg 12 hourly.

8

Antituberculous drugs

FIRST LINE AGENTS

Currently recommended first-line therapy for pulmonary TB, includes a combination of isoniazid, rifampicin and ethambutol together to prevent emergence of resistant mycobacteria. Ethambutol is usually stopped after two months and two other drugs are continued for a total of nine months, although shorter courses are under investigation. Courses of 12 months are currently used for treatment of extrapulmonary tuberculosis.

ISONIAZID

Activity
Bactericidal to *M. tuberculosis*. Active only against mycobacteria.

Principal uses
Treatment and prophylaxis of TB.

Administration

Adults
Oral/IM: 300 mg daily (approx 3 mg/kg/day).

Children
6 mg/kg daily.

For treatment of miliary disease or TB meningitis give 10 mg/kg/day in 3 divided doses.

Isoniazid is excreted renally as free drug and metabolites. It is efficiently absorbed following oral administration and is well distributed to tissue and CSF.

Fifty to sixty per cent of Europeans are slow acetylators and are more prone to pyridoxine deficiency. Acetylation is slowest in Caucasians and Blacks.

Isoniazid for prophylaxis of TB:
Recommended for close child contacts of TB. Probably also of value for patients with a history of TB who subsequently require high doses of immunosuppressive drugs.

Adults
300 mg daily for 12 months.

Children
5 mg/kg daily for 12 months.
Some authorities believe that prophylaxis of immunosuppressed patients should continue for life or until immunosuppressants are stopped.

Principal side effects
Nauseas, vomiting, rashes. Peripheral neuritis with high doses (this may be avoided by giving 20–50 mg pyridoxine daily). Rarely: pellagra, psychosis, thrombocytopenia. Hepatitis rarely—risk is greatest in older patients with pre-existing liver disease.

RIFAMPICIN

Activity
Broad-spectrum activity against staphylococci, Gram-negative bacilli, haemophilus, meningococci and bacteroides, but resistance develops rapidly during use when given alone for treatment of acute pyogenic infections, because of the selection of mutants insensitive to rifampicin. Actively bactericidal against mycobacteria.

Principal uses
1. Tuberculosis. (NB: It is best to avoid rifampicin initially if trials of therapy of suspected TB are undertaken, because its activity against a wide range of pathogens may obscure diagnosis.)
2. Severe staphylococcal infections such as meningitis or endocarditis, if other agents are unsuitable, in combination with another antistaphylococcal agent (do not use alone because resistance develops readily). The microbiologist should test the sensitivity of a combination against a particular isolate to ensure that there is no antagonism.
3. Prophylaxis of meningococcal meningitis (see p. 85).

Administration

Adults
Oral: 450–600 mg daily (before food) (approximately 10 mg/kg body weight).

Children
Oral: 10–20 mg/kg/day.

Intravenous rifampicin is available from the manufacturers but is not marketed in the UK. Preparations combining rifampicin and isoniazid are available to simplify medication for TB patients. Rifampicin is mainly eliminated in bile, therefore dosage adjustments are not needed in renal impairment. It should be used with care in patients with liver disease. Rifampicin diffuses readily into tissues and CSF.

Principal side effects
Red urine, tears and sputum (because of ready diffusion). Rashes, jaundice, gastro-intestinal disturbances. Intermittent treatment may cause the 'flu syndrome'. Rifampicin may induce liver enzymes, inactivating other drugs, e.g. steroids, contraceptive pill, anticoagulants. Contra-indicated in pregnancy, because of possible teratogenicity. Thrombocytopenic purpura. Allergic nephritis.

ETHAMBUTOL

Activity
Static antimycobacterial activity.

Principal uses
Usually given during initial phase of therapy (for 2 months or until results of sensitivity tests are known) in combination with isoniazid and rifampicin (or streptomycin).

Administration

Adults
Oral: 15 mg/kg/day. 25 mg/kg/day may be needed for re-treatment, or if only one other agent is being used and in treatment of TB meningitis.

Children
Safety in young children not established.

Reduced dosage is needed in renal failure and serum levels should be monitored—'trough' levels should not exceed 3 mg/1.

Principal side effects

Optic neuritis—dose related; not usually associated with lower dosage (15 mg/kg/day) in the absence of renal failure. First signs of optic neuritis are often changes in colour vision, usually reversible if the drug is withdrawn. Nevertheless, permanent blindness may occur.

Do not give to young children and avoid, or use with great care, in the elderly.

STREPTOMYCIN

Activity

Broad-spectrum bactericidal activity against coliforms and staphylococci. Bactericidal against mycobacteria (activity is greater than other aminoglycosides).

Principal uses

In treatment of TB when a first line drug is contra-indicated or not tolerated.

Administration

Adults

IM: 1 g daily. Over 40 years: 750 mg daily. Some patients need only 500 mg daily.

Children

IM: 30 mg/kg/24 hours. Up to 1 g daily.

Serum levels in the elderly or in renal impairment should be monitored in order to adjust dosage (pre-dose levels should not exceed 3 mg/l).

Principal side effects

Ototoxicity (deafness).

SECOND LINE AGENTS

Agents to use against strains resistant to first line drugs. Resistance in European strains of *M. tuberculosis* remains uncommon, but is higher in strains from Africa and the Far East.

PARA-AMINOSALICYLATE

Activity
Not as active as other agents against mycobacteria and so large doses are required.

Principal uses
Tuberculosis resistant to other agents.

Administration

Adults
Oral: 8–15 g daily as divided doses.

Principal side effects
As for salicylates. Nausea is very common, leading to poor compliance. Hypersensitivity, rashes. Avoid in renal impairment.

PYRAZINAMIDE

Cidal antimycobacterial activity. Good penetration into CSF and therefore useful in TB meningitis.

Administration
Oral: 500 mg 8 hourly (no more than 3 g daily or 20–30 mg/kg daily in 3 doses).

Principal side effects:
Hepatotoxicity.

CYCLOSERINE

Weak activity against mycobacteria in vitro, but effective, in vivo. Broad-spectrum antibacterial activity, including staphylococci and coliforms.
Mycobacteria resistant to streptomycin and isoniazid are usually sensitive to cycloserine.

Administration

Adults

Oral: 250 mg every 12 hours, increasing to 250 mg every 8 hours.

Principal side effects

Neurotoxic; headaches, dizziness, depression, excitability.

CAPREOMYCIN

Active against streptomycin-resistant *M. tuberculosis*.

Administration

Adults

IM: 1 g daily.

Principal side effects

Hypersensitivity, e.g. rashes, urticaria. Hepatotoxicity, ototoxicity. Renal damage.

9

Antifungal agents

AMPHOTERICIN B

Polyenes such as amphotericin and nystatin are antifungal agents derived from streptomyces bacteria; their activity is due to binding to the fungal cell membrane, leading to disruption of the organism.

The only polyene which may be given parenterally, amphotericin is probably still the most useful drug for systemic fungal infections in spite of its potential toxicity. Penetration into body fluids is relatively poor.

Activity
Fungicidal against candida, histoplasma, coccidioides, cryptococcus and aspergillus.

Principal uses
1. Topical application for mucosal infections caused by candida.
2. Treatment of systemic fungal infections—systemic candidiasis, histoplasmosis, coccidioidomycosis, cryptococcal meningitis, aspergillosis, mucormycosis. Surgery is usually required for removal of aspergilloma.
3. Amoebic meningitis.

Administration
1. Oral—Treatment of oral candidiasis or to reduce colonisation load in immunosuppressed patients where systemic dissemination is a risk. Tablets/lozenges/suspension—100–200 mg 6 hourly.
2. Pessary, for vaginal candidiasis: 50–100 mg at night for 14 nights.
3. Intravenous amphotericin—Give as continuous infusion in 5% dextrose at concentration not exceeding 0.1 mg/ml. Doses should be built up gradually to minimise toxicity. Give initial test dose of 1 mg in 20 ml 5% dextrose, then 5 mg, 15 mg, 25 mg, on subsequent days. Although maintenance doses of 1 mg/kg/day, or even

1.5 mg/kg/day may be given, toxicity may be minimised by keeping doses at 0.6 mg/kg/day, if necessary giving the drug on alternate days; combination with flucytosine may permit smaller effective doses of amphotericin to be used (amphotericin enhances penetration of flucytosine into fungal cells, producing synergy). In severely ill patients, doses may be built up from 1 mg to 0.25 mg/kg/day to 0.5 mg/kg/day on a daily basis.

4. Intrathecal amphotericin—small intrathecal doses may be required for treatment of meningitis since penetration into CSF following intravenous administration is poor.

Principal side effects
Nephrotoxicity is virtually invariable (but amphotericin may be given cautiously in renal impairment if necessary because the drug is probably metabolised; excretion through the kidneys is slow and incomplete). Renal function usually recovers after stopping treatment, albeit sometimes after several months. Phlebitis at infusion site. Fever, rigors, nausea. Hypokalaemia. Cardiac arrhythmias.

NYSTATIN

A polyene too toxic for parenteral use, but very poorly absorbed after ingestion. It is used locally to control candida infections in mouth and vagina.

Activity
Greatest activity against yeast-like fungi (such as candida), which are invariably sensitive. It has no activity against filamentous fungi or histoplasma.

Administration

Tablets
1 tablet (500 000 units) every 6 hours or 2 tablets in severe infections.

Pessary
100 000 units per pessary. Insert 1 or 2 per vaginam each night for 14 nights.

Principal site effects
Nausea, vomiting.

FLUCYTOSINE

A synthetic fluorinated pyrimidine which interferes with fungal nucleic acid synthesis; good penetration into tissue and body fluids including CSF and urine.

Activity
Fungistatic against candida, cryptococcus, other yeasts. Resistance may exist de novo, or may develop rapidly during therapy. Sensitivity must be tested using specialised techniques. Use in combination with amphotericin may prevent emergence of resistance to flucytosine. No activity against filamentous fungi. It should not be used alone in treatment of serious fungal infection because of the potential acquisition of resistance.

Administration
Well absorbed after oral administration, but may also be given intravenously.

Adults
Oral/IV: 25–50 mg/kg 6 hourly.

Children
Oral/IV: 25–50 mg/ 6 hourly.

Principal side effects
Nausea, vomiting, rashes. Thrombocytopenia, neutropenia, jaundice. Toxicity is usually dose-related: serum levels should be measured in patients with impaired renal function. Weekly blood counts should be monitored if treatment is prolonged.

IMIDAZOLES

Synthetic agents with broad-spectrum antifungal activity.

CLOTRIMAZOLE

Clotrimazole is available only for topical use mainly because of toxicity associated with systemic administration.

Activity
Candida, dermatophytes, trichomonas.

Principal uses
Local candidiasis or ringworm. Vaginal infection caused by candida and/or trichomonas.

Administration
1. 1% cream—apply to skin 2-3 times daily until 2 weeks after clinical cure.
2. Vaginal tablet—100 mg at night for 6 nights or 200 mg at night for 3 nights.
3. Vaginal cream—apply 5 g twice daily for 3 days or once nightly for 6 nights.

Principal side effect
Local irritation.

MICONAZOLE

An imidazole which may be given locally, by mouth or by the intravenous route. Absorption after oral administration is incomplete and therapeutic serum levels are difficult to maintain. It should not be given with amphotericin because of possible antagonism.

Activity
Yeasts, dermatophytes, broad-spectrum antifungal activity, but less active against aspergillus.

Principal uses
Local candidiasis. Dermatophyte infections. Systemic fungal infections which are not life-threatening (where amphotericin would probably be treatment of choice). It should not be used in urinary tract infections because of inadequate levels in urine.

Administration
1. Oral: 250 mg 6 hourly or 5-10 ml oral gel 6 hourly.
2. Topical application: as 2% cream or powder for ringworm—apply morning and evening.
3. Vaginal pessaries: 200 mg for 7 nights.
4. Intravenous—*Adults*: 600 mg 8 hourly. *Children*: 40 mg/kg/day.

Principal side effects
Nausea, vomiting, especially at high dosage. Pruritis, rashes. Phlebitis when given intravenously.

ECONAZOLE

An analogue of miconazole used topically in treatment of cutaneous or mucosal candidiasis.

KETOCONAZOLE

A newer, as yet incompletely evaluated imidazole for oral administration, with the advantage of better absorption from the gastro-intestinal tract than miconazole.

Principal uses
Superficial fungal infections caused by yeasts and dermatophytes. Its value in systemic fungal infections is still to be assessed further. It may be a useful prophylactic in immunosuppressed patients at risk of disseminated candidiasis.

Administration

Adults
Oral: 200 mg daily with food increasing to 400 mg daily in severe infection.

Children
Oral: 3 mg/kg/24 hours.

Principal side effects
Rarely nausea, rashes, pruritis, hepatitis.

OTHER ANTIFUNGAL AGENTS

GRISEOFULVIN

Inactive topically, but is absorbed from the gastro-intestinal tract and concentrated in keratin.

Activity
Active against dermatophytes.

Principal uses
Severe dermatophyte infections.

Administration

Adults
Oral: 500 mg–1 g daily (divided doses or every 24 hrs).

Children
Oral: 10 mg/kg/day.

Duration of treatment—ringworm of skin and hair 4–6 weeks, nails up to 12 months.

Principal side effects
Headache, nausea, rashes. Do not use in pregnancy, liver failure or porphyria.

10

Antiprotozoal agents

ANTIMALARIAL AGENTS

CHLOROQUINE

Activity

A 4-aminoquinolone active against the asexual erythrocyte forms but not exoerythrocytic tissue forms of plasmodia. *P. vivax, P. ovale* and *P. malariae* are invariably sensitive. Strains of *P. falciparum* resistant to chloroquine are becoming increasingly common in E. Africa, S.E. Asia and Central and South America. The distribution of chloroquine resistance is changing rapidly. Chloroquine is also active against amoebae.

Principal uses

1. Treatment of choice in benign tertian malaria (usually caused by *P. vivax.*) May be used in treatment of malignant tertian malaria acquired in areas where resistance is not known.
2. Malaria prophylaxis for zones where resistance in *P. falciparum* is not a problem. Some authorities claim that prophylactic use of chloroquine should be abandoned because of the possibility of promoting chloroquine resistance. However, it is preferred by others for short-term prophylaxis because the risk of malaria breakthrough is less than with proguanil, in areas where chloroquine resistance is not a problem.

Administration

Treatment of malaria
Oral: initially 600 mg followed by a further 300 mg after 6 hrs then 150 mg 12 hourly for a further 2 days.
IM/IV: may be used if vomiting or coma (in *P. falciparum* malaria) make oral therapy impossible. Give initial 200–300 mg parenterally followed by oral therapy or a second injection after 6 hours. Do not

give by intravenous route to infants because of possible cardiovascular toxicity.

Principal side effects
Headaches, nausea, vomiting, diarrhoea, rashes. Prolonged high dosage may lead to corneal or retinal damage. Side effects associated with regular use of chloroquine make proguanil more suitable than chloroquine for long-term prophylaxis, i.e. more than 2 or 3 years.

QUININE SULPHATE

A chinochona alkaloid.

Activity
Destroys asexual erythrocytic forms of plasmodia including chloroquine-resistant *P. falciparum*.

Principal uses
Emergency treatment of cerebral malaria due to *P. falciparum*, or severe infections caused by chloroquine-resistant strains, or in patients failing to respond to chloroquine.

Administration
Oral: 600 mg 8 hourly for at least 4 doses.
IV: 5–10 mg/kg over 4 hours for 4 doses spaced at 12–24 hour intervals (dose determined by size of patient, severity of illness and presence of liver disease). Total dose should not exceed 500 mg.

Principal side effects
Chinchonism—tinnitus, headache, nausea, abdominal pain, visual disturbances, blindness, hypersentivity.

PRIMAQUINE PHOSPHATE

An 8-aminoquinolone.

Activity
Active against exo-erythrocytic forms of *P. vivax* and *P. falciparum*.

Principal uses
Eradication of tissue forms in benign tertian malaria following initial treatment with chloroquine or quinine.

Administration

Adults
Oral: 15 mg daily for 14 days.

Children
Oral: 7.5 mg daily for 14 days.

Principal side effects
Anorexia, nausea, vomiting, jaundice. Less often: marrow depression, haemolytic anaemia.
Caution—haemolysis in patients with glucose-6-phosphate dehydrogenase deficiency is precipitated by primaquine.

MALARIA CHEMOPROPHYLAXIS

The problem of malaria prophylaxis is becoming increasingly difficult because of the changing resistance patterns of malarial parasites. Current recommendations may be obtained from the School of Hygiene and Tropical Medicine, London. Tel: 01–636–8636.

Chloroquine, proguanil or pyrimethamine are used traditionally for malaria prophylaxis, but may no longer be effective for travellers in S.E. Asia, E. Africa and Central and Southern America because of resistance in *P. falciparum*. In general there is cross-resistance between chloroquine, proguanil and pyrimethamine but some chloroquine-sensitive plasmodia may be resistant to proguanil and pyrimethamine. Travellers to areas where chloroquine resistance is recognised should take Maloprim or Fansidar (sulpha/pyrimethamine combinations).

Malaria prohylaxis should start one week before departure (or 24 hours before when taking daily tablets) and continue for four to six weeks after leaving malarial zones. Other protective measures such as mosquito nets and insect repellents must also be remembered.

CHLOROQUINE

Administration

Adults
300 mg weekly for prophylaxis (except S. and C. America, S.E. Africa and E. Africa).

Children
1–5 years: 150 mg weekly.

6–12 years: 225 mg weekly.

Infants
75 mg weekly.

PROGUANIL

The agent most commonly used in malaria prophylaxis although there is resistance in *P. falciparum* in East Africa and Madagascar, as well as foci of resistance in S.E. Asia and Central and Southern America. It is best avoided in these areas. Like chloroquine, it is safe for infants and in pregnancy.

Administration

Adults
Oral: 100–200 mg daily (a daily dosage may be more easily remembered than a weekly regimen as for chloroquine). The higher dosage is required in sub-Saharan Africa.

Children
Oral: <6 years 50 mg daily (½ tablet). 6–12 years 75 mg daily (¾ tablet).

Start prophylaxis one week before travelling to endemic area and continue for 4 weeks after return (in practice, protective levels are achieved if prophylaxis is started only one day before departure, but it is useful to become accustomed to taking the drug regularly).

Principal side effects

Rarely, vomiting, epigastric pain, haematuria.

PYRIMETHAMINE

A folate antagonist which may be used for malaria prophylaxis in zones where chloroquine-resistant *P. falciparum* is not a problem. It has the advantage of being tasteless (both proguanil and chloroquine taste bitter). Pyrimethamine breakthrough is reported to be more likely than failure of proguanil.

Administration

Adults
25 mg weekly.

Children
Avoid under the age of 5 years.

Principal side effects
Depression of haemopoeisis with prolonged treatment.

MALOPRIM

A combination of pyrimethamine 12.5 mg and dapsone 100 mg.

Principal uses
For prophylaxis of malaria for travellers to areas where chloroquine resistance is recognised. At present Maloprim is considered acceptable for use by pregnant women visiting areas where chloroquine or proguanil resistance makes use of these drugs potentially unsafe. Theoretical risks of foetal damage due to interference with folate metabolism must be weighed against the importance of reliable malaria prophylaxis.

Administration

Adults
One tablet weekly. Optimal dose may in future be raised to 2 tablets weekly.

Children
Not recommended under 5 years.

Principal side effects
As for sulphonamides. Maloprim may be given to individuals allergic to sulphonamides provided there is no cross-allergenicity to sulphones. Probably advisable to give folate supplements if used in pregnancy.

FANSIDAR

A combination of pyrimethamine 25 mg and sulphadoxine 500 mg.

Principal uses
Malaria prophylaxis in areas where there may be resistance to chloroquine. It may also be used for treatment of chloroquine-resistant malaria. Fansidar resistance has now emerged as a problem in Thailand.

Administration
One tablet weekly.

Principal side effects
Sulphonamide sensitivity. Avoid in pregnancy and the neonatal period.

11

Antihelmintics

Expert advice is often needed in treatment of worm infestations and may be obtained from the London School of Hygiene and Tropical Medicine (Tel: 01–636–8636) or local infectious diseases units.

TREATMENT OF THREADWORM AND ROUNDWORM INFESTATIONS

PIPERAZINE

Activity
Active against threadworm (*Enterobius vermicularis*) and roundworm (*Ascaris lumbricoides*). A cheap and effective drug but now largely superseded, at least in wealthier societies, by newer but more expensive agents such as mebendazole, because of occasional but severe neurotoxic reactions which may occur with piperazine.

Principal side effects
Rarely causes gastro-intestinal disturbances, skin rashes and neurotoxicity. Contra-indicated in epilepsy and renal/hepatic impairment.

MEBENDAZOLE

Activity
Active against threadworm, roundworm, hookworm and whipworm.

Administration (as tablets or suspension)
Threadworm: Treat patient and all members of the family to prevent re-infection. Give 100 mg weekly for 6 consecutive weeks.
Whipworm: 100 mg 12 hourly for 3 days.
Roundworm: 100 mg 12 hourly for 3 days.
Hookworm: 100 mg 12 hourly for 3 days.

Caution: Do not use in pregnancy or in children less than 2 yrs.

Principal side effects
Abdominal pain and diarrhoea reported rarely.

THIABENDAZOLE

Activity and principal uses
Active against ascaris, whipworm, threadworm, hookworm, strongyloides. Useful in patients with mixed infestations. The only antihelmintic drug which is absorbed from the gut and produces activity both in the intestine and in tissue. It is therefore the treatment of choice for *Strongyloides stercoralis* whose larvae migrate into tissue.

Administration
For strongyloides: 25 mg/kg twice daily for 3 days (maximum 3 g per day).

Principal side effects
Anorexia, vomiting, headache, dizziness, diarrhoea, hypersensitivity. Caution in renal/hepatic impairment.

TREATMENT OF TAPEWORM INFESTATION

NICLOSAMIDE

Activity
Active against *Taenia saginata*, *T. solium* and *Diphyllobothrium latum* (the fish tapeworm), and *Hymenolepis nana* (dwarf tapeworm).

Principal use
Tapeworm infestation.

Administration
Taenia: 2 g chewed and swallowed with a little water on an empty stomach then followed by a purgative after 2 hours.

Hymenolepis nana: Dwarf tapeworm infestation involves multiplication of the parasite within the intestinal villi, and therefore longer courses are required—2 g is given on the first day followed by 1 g daily for the next 6 days. Repeat one month later. Hymenolepis infections however rarely give rise to symptoms and treatment is not usually required.

Principal side effects
Gastro-intestinal upsets. Pruritis.

Caution—For treatment of *T. solium* (pig tapeworm, now rare in the UK) refer to a specialist unit because entire adult worm and ova must be eliminated in order to avoid cystercercosis. Niclosamide may cause release of *T. solium* ova in the intestine, with subsequent risk of cystercercosis, but to minimise this possibility an anti-emetic may be given 1 hour before the dose, and a purgative 2 hours later.

TREATMENT OF HOOKWORM INFESTATION

BEPHENIUM HYDROXYNAPHTHOATE

Active against both species of hookworm (*A. duodenale* and *N. americanus*), although because of reduced potency against *N. americanus* it is no longer the drug of choice for hookworm infestation.

Also kills ascaris and trichostrongylus. Very little is absorbed from the gut.

Administration

Adults and children over 2 years
Single dose of 2.5 g sachet in water whilst fasting (no food for 2 hours).

Principal side effects
Nausea, vomiting.

MEBENDAZOLE

This drug has activity not only against hookworm but also against other worms (see p. 80), an advantage in tropical countries where patients often have multiple infestations.

PYRANTEL

Also an effective broad-spectrum anti-helmintic; a single dose of 10 mg/kg is repeated after 48 h.

TREATMENT OF SCHISTOSOMIASIS

NIRIDAZOLE

Activity
Active against *Schistosoma haematobium* and *S. mansoni*. Response

less satisfactory for *S. japonicum*—and should not be used for this infestation, where liver damage is more common.

Principal use
Bilharzia infection. The drug of choice for *S. haematobium* infection.

Administration
Oral: 25 mg/kg daily in 2 doses for 7 days.

Principal side effects
Gastro-intestinal irritation. Neurological toxicity—convulsions, psychosis—may occur if venous anastomoses in portal hypertension allow the drug to by-pass the liver and so avoid conjugation. Liver damage may complicate *S. mansoni* or *S. japonicum* infestation and niridazole should be avoided if there is evidence of liver disease, since it is metabolised by the liver.

OXAMNIQUINE

A quinolone, which is the treatment of choice for *S. mansoni* infection, but whose activity against *S. haematobium* is limited.
    20 mg/kg is given daily for 1–3 days

PRAZIQUANTEL

A new drug found to be safe and effective with activity against all three species of human schistosomes. It is given as a single oral dose of 50 mg/kg. Side effects are mild, most commonly abdominal discomfort, giddiness and fever (possibly due to a reaction to dead parasites rather than direct drug toxicity).

12

Antibiotic prophylaxis

Ideally, antibiotic prophylaxis should be used only where it is indispensible and of proven value. The infection to be prevented should be caused by a single bacterial species which is invariably sensitive to the drug, and which has little tendency to develop resistance to it. The drug should be free of serious side effects, at least in the manner in which it is employed for prophylaxis. Prophylaxis of a number of conditions discussed below largely fulfils these conditions but, of late, empirical broad-spectrum prophylactic regimes have been successful in preventing infection following surgery, notably colo-rectal procedures, where a range of potential pathogens may be implicated.

PROPHYLAXIS WHERE A NARROW SPECTRUM ANTIBIOTIC IS GIVEN TO PREVENT AN INFECTION BY A KNOWN PATHOGEN

Prevention of recurrent rheumatic fever in children
Penicillin V: 125–250 mg 12 hourly (oral).
In penicillin allergy—sulphadimidine 500 mg–1 g daily (oral), or erythromycin.

Prevention of endocarditis in patients with heart valve lesions
Given when patients with valvular heart disease undergo dental manipulations or other procedures likely to cause bacteraemia.
1. For patients who do not have valve prosthesis:
Amoxycillin: single 3 g oral dose 1 hour before extraction.
or, for penicillin-hypersensitive patients, or those already on penicillin for rheumatic fever prophylaxis, who may be colonised by penicillin-resistant bacteria:
Erythromycin: 1.5 g oral dose (stearate) 60 minutes before procedure, then 500 mg after 6 hours.

2. For patients with valve prosthesis or undergoing urogenital procedures or gut surgery, where a wider range of potential pathogens (including *Streptococcus faecalis*) may be implicated:
Amoxycillin 1 g IM (in 2.5 ml of 1% lignocaine) *plus* gentamicin 120 mg IM 30 minutes before procedure. Give 500 mg amoxycillin by mouth or by injection 6 hours later.

In penicillin-allergic patients, vancomycin 1 g IV should be substituted for amoxycillin.

Prevention of clostridial gas gangrene in patients undergoing amputation of ischaemic limbs or with contaminated traumatic wounds

Benzylpenicillin 300–600 mg by intramuscular injection 6 hourly, starting with pre-med and continuing for 5 days, *or* procaine penicillin 2.4 g every 12 hours for 5 days *or* metronidazole 500 mg IV at induction of anaesthesia then 400 mg orally 8 hourly for 5 days.

Prevention of meningitis is contacts of patients with meningococcal infection

Prophylaxis is indicated for household members of patients with meningococcal infection, and for medical staff who have been in very close contact (e.g. mouth-to-mouth resuscitation). Present evidence suggests a combination (to prevent emergence of resistance):
Minocycline 200 mg 12 hourly *plus* rifampicin 600 mg 12 hourly for 48 hours for adults.

NB Vertigo is an important side-effect of minocycline and all those taking the drug should be warned of this possibility.

For children alternatives are:
Rifampicin alone:
>12 years: 600 mg 12 hourly
1–12 years: 10 mg/kg 12 hourly
3–12 months: 5 mg/kg 12 hourly.
or
A sulphonamide, when strain is known to be sensitive to sulphonamides:
>12 years: 1 g 12 hourly
1–12 years: 500 mg 12 hourly
3–12 months: 250 mg 12 hourly.

Rifampicin should be avoided in pregnancy and sulphonamides in the last trimester.

Prevention for contacts of diphtheria

For close contacts, in conjunction with immunisation of susceptible individuals:

Adults
Erythromycin 500 mg (oral) 6 hourly for 5 days.

Children
Erythromycin 125–500 mg (oral) 6 hourly for 5 days.

Prevention of tetanus in contaminated traumatic wounds

Surgical debridement and toxoid, sometimes with antitoxin are most important; the role of antibiotic prophylaxis is not proven, but chemoprophylaxis is recommended in some circumstances.

The most reliable prophylaxis is probably fortified procaine penicillin 300 mg 12 hourly (intramuscular) for 5 days for high-risk patients. Erythromycin or metronidazole are suitable alternatives.

Malaria

(see p. 76)

Tuberculosis

(see p. 63)

PROPHYLAXIS WHERE A VARIETY OF POTENTIAL PATHOGENS MUST BE CONSIDERED

Prophylaxis of certain potentially contaminated surgical procedures has been found to be effective in preventing postoperative sepsis, although a wide range of bacteria must be considered as potential pathogens. There is a risk that antibiotic-resistant bacteria may emerge, so it is essential that such courses be *as short as possible*. Bacteraemia and seeding of organisms are most likely to occur at the time of surgery, and so it is important that antibiotic levels in tissue should be high at the time of operation and in the *immediate* postoperative period. (It is of course well recognised that antimicrobial prophylaxis can never be a substitute for careful surgical technique. Peroperative prophylaxis cannot for example prevent infection resulting from anastomotic leakage). Prophylaxis should never give rise to a false sense of security or detract from the need for scrupulous aseptic technique.

Colo-rectal surgery

Metronidazole 500 mg IV over 20–30 minutes at induction of anaesthesia, followed by 2 further doses of 1 g by suppository at 8 hourly intervals (or 500 mg IV, if the rectal route must be avoided).

Plus gentamicin 80–120 mg IV at induction then 2 further doses of 80 mg at 8 hourly intervals (dose and interval may need to be adjusted according to renal function). (*Or* cefuroxime 750 mg IV at induction, then 2 further doses of 750 mg IV or IM at 8 hourly intervals, in place of gentamicin).

Full therapeutic courses of 5 days or more must be given to patients with *established* infection, e.g. gangrenous appendicitis. There is some evidence that metronidazole alone produces results as good as a combination of metronidazole and gentamicin. The need for gentamicin to prevent Gram-negative aerobic infection is still uncertain. Mechanical bowel preparation is important in elective colonic surgery.

Biliary surgery
Some surgeons reserve prophylaxis for selected patients who are at special risk of infection, (e.g. jaundiced or elderly patients or those with biliary stones):
Cefuroxime 750 mg IV at induction (or IM with pre-med).

Gastric surgery
Prophylaxis is used to 'cover' resections and other procedures carrying a high risk of infection:
Cefuroxime 750 mg IV at induction (or IM with pre-med) *plus* further 750 mg IV/IM 8 hours later.

Vaginal hysterectomy
Metronidazole 500 mg IV over 20–30 minutes at induction of anaesthesia *plus* further 1 g suppository after 8 hours.

Hip replacement
Benefits apply to patients operated on in conventional theatres (i.e. not ultra-clean air systems):
Cefuroxime 1.5 g IV at induction, followed by further 1.5 g IV or IM at 8 and 16 hours.

Open-heart surgery
Antibiotic-resistant opportunists may be a problem so a combination is employed:
Cloxacillin 500 mg plus
Benzylpenicillin 600 mg plus
Gentamicin (dose according to age, weight and renal function).

Give loading dose IM with pre-med then IV booster at end of cardio-pulmonary by-pass, then IV bolus doses at appropriate intervals over the next 48 hours.

Vancomycin or cefuroxime are suggested for penicillin-allergic patients in place of cloxacillin and penicillin.

Urological surgery
Prophlaxis of certain procedures where risk of bacteraemia is high, e.g. transrectal biopsy of prostate, difficult urethral dilatation:
Gentamicin 80–120 mg IV at induction, *plus* 2 further doses of 80 mg at appropriate intervals postoperatively (depending on renal function).

Or a suitable antibiotic as indicated by in vitro tests if a urinary tract pathogen has been cultured. In such cases full therapeutic courses should be given.

It is important to recognise that these recommendations may be modified in the light of further experience of their use.

13

Laboratory control of antimicrobial therapy

Serum levels of an antibiotic with a low therapeutic-to-toxic ratio should be monitored to make sure that therapeutic concentrations are achieved and to check that the drug is being eliminated and potentially toxic levels avoided.

Assay of aminoglycosides is an important aspect of management of patients treated with these antibiotics. Monitoring of antibiotic serum levels is necessary for patients with impaired renal function or in whom recommended doses do not appear to be controlling infection. It is usually advisable to perform assays after 24 to 48 hours therapy in seriously ill patients or the elderly and to repeat subsequently as required. Serum levels should also be checked in patients who have received an aminoglycoside for more than one week, in whom progressive accumulation may occur, and in neonates whose handling of the drugs may be unpredictable. Other drugs may require monitoring to avoid dose-related toxicity, especially in renal impairment, and include chloramphenicol in babies, ethambutol and flucytosine. Penicillin and erythromycin levels should be measured in patients with renal impairment who require treatment in high dosage. Other antibiotics may be monitored if clinically indicated, particularly in serious infections treated with oral antibiotics, (such as tuberculosis) where a poor response may result from inadequate absorption of antibiotic.

Always discuss your intention to request antibiotic assays with the laboratory and state clearly the time of blood samples in relation to the doses given. Blood should be sampled at times to coincide with peak and trough levels, i.e. for most drugs, 60 minutes post injection (IM or IV) for peaks and immediately preceding a dose for troughs. It is important to state whether other antibiotics are being given concurrently or have been taken recently.

INTERPRETATION OF RESULTS

Individuals may vary in their pharmacokinetic handling of drugs. Interpretation of results and subsequent dose adjustment is achieved by consideration of both clinical and laboratory aspects of individual patients: medical microbiologists should work closely with clinicians in the control of antimicrobial therapy.

BACTERICIDAL ACTIVITY OF SERUM

It is important to ensure that antimicrobial therapy of patients with infective endocarditis produces fully bactericidal activity in serum. This is especially important if oral treatment is used after initial parenteral therapy; it is essential to ensure that sufficient drug is absorbed. Therapy is considered adequate if a patient's serum remains bactericidal at a dilution of 1 in 8 or more against the organism isolated from blood culture. Blood should be taken just before a dose and also at a time to coincide with the peak post-dose level. The laboratory should be notified the day before this test is required since an overnight culture of the organism must be prepared.

MINIMUM INHIBITORY CONCENTRATIONS OF ANTIBIOTICS

Disc sensitivity tests are designed to produce a convenient but usually reliable prediction of the therapeutic activity of a range of antibiotics against clinical isolates. Sometimes it is necessary to measure the susceptibility of an organism more accurately. The minimum inhibitory concentration (MIC) of an antibiotic is the smallest concentration of antibiotic which will inhibit growth of an organism.

The minimum bactericidal concentration (MBC) is the smallest concentration of antibiotic which will kill the organism. These tests are done as part of the investigation of the activity of new drugs and may also be undertaken in clinical bacteriology laboratories, for example to determine the MIC and MBC of penicillin to an isolate from a patient with infective endocarditis, since disc tests cannot detect small increases in resistance, which may be important in the treatment of serious infections. Higher doses of antibiotics are needed for the treatment of infection caused by less susceptible bacteria.

TESTS OF COMBINED ANTIBACTERIAL ACTION

If two drugs are being used in the treatment of serious infections (for example flucloxacillin and fusidic acid in staphylococcal endocarditis) it is often worthwhile investigating their interaction against a clinical isolate. A combination showing in vitro antagonism should be avoided. It is useful to be able to use two drugs which show synergy.

14

Antibiotic use in renal and hepatic failure

RENAL FAILURE

Patients with impaired renal function should receive the recommended initial drug dose, unless the antibiotic has a very narrow toxic/therapeutic ratio; for example aminoglycosides, whose initial dosage may be determined by nomogram or by data sheet recommendations. Thereafter dosage should either be reduced and/or the interval between doses lengthened according to the results of serum assays.

Table 14.1 shows the dosage recommendations for antibiotics in patients with renal impairment, based on their serum half-lives.

Antimicrobials which should be *avoided* in renal failure include the following:

Tetracyclines (except doxycycline)
Chloramphenicol
Cephaloridine, cephalothin
Nitrofurantoin
Nalidixic acid
PAS
Ampicillin esters e.g. talampicillin

HEPATIC FAILURE

Drugs metabolised or detoxified by the liver should in general be prescribed in reduced dosage, with monitoring of serum levels. These drugs include:

Chloramphenicol   Nalidixic acid
Tetracycline   Isoniazid
Erythromycin estolate   Pyrazinamide
Clindamycin   Rifampicin
Fusidic acid   Niridazole
Nitrofurantoin

Table 14.1 Antibiotic use in renal failure

Guidelines for dosage in renal failure (in management of serious infection, where dosage is critical, therapy should be controlled by measurement of serum antibiotic levels)

Drug	Major elimination routes	GFR > 50 ml/min	GFR 10–50 ml/min	GFR < 10 ml/min	Effect of haemodialysis	Remarks
Group I: Normal dosage in renal failure						
Erythromycin	Hepatic	Unchanged	Unchanged	Unchanged except when high doses are used (e.g. Legionnaires' disease)	Removed slowly or not at all	May be ototoxic when given in *large doses* to patients in renal failure
Sodium fusidate	Hepatic	Unchanged	Unchanged	Unchanged		
Rifampicin	Hepatic	Unchanged	Unchanged	Unchanged	? Not removed	May rarely cause acute renal failure
Group II: Minor dosage adjustments						
Penicillins:						
Benzylpenicillin	Renal (hepatic)	Dose unchanged 8 hourly dose	No dose reduction 8 hourly dose	Reduce dose by 50% Give 8–12 hourly. Max. 6 g daily. Serum penicillin levels should be measured when high doses are used in renal failure	Removed by haemodialysis	Monitor serum electrolytes

Table 14.1 (*cont'd*)

Guidelines for dosage in renal failure (in management of serious infection, where dosage is critical, therapy should be controlled by measurement of serum antibiotic levels)

Drug	Major elimination routes	GFR > 50 ml/min	GFR 10–50 ml/min	GFR < 10 ml/min	Effect of haemodialysis	Remarks
Ampicillin	Renal (hepatic)	No dose reduction Give 6 hourly	No dose reduction Give 9 hourly	No dose reduction Give 12 hourly	Removed by haemodialysis	
Amoxycillin	Renal	No dose reduction Give 8 hourly	No dose reduction Give 12 hourly	No dose reduction Give 16 hourly	Removed by haemodialysis	
Cloxacillin Flucloxacillin	Hepatic (renal)	No dose reduction Give 6 hourly	No dose reduction Give 6 hourly	No dose reduction Give 8 hourly	Not removed by haemodialysis	
Carbenicillin	Renal (hepatic)	No dose reduction Give 6 hourly	Reduce dose to 75% Give 12 hourly	Reduce dose to 25–50% Give 12 hourly	Removed by haemodialysis	Monitor serum sodium because of Na load. Give recommended dose after haemodialysis
Mezlocillin	Renal	No dose reduction Give 8 hourly	No dose reduction Give 8 hourly	No dose reduction Give 12 hourly	Removed by haemodialysis	Monitor serum sodium because of Na load. Give recommended dose after haemodialysis
Azlocillin	Renal	No dose reduction Give 8 hourly	No dose reduction Give 8 hourly	No dose reduction Give 12 hourly	Removed by haemodialysis	Monitor serum sodium because of Na load. Give recommended dose after haemodialysis

Cephalosporins: Cephalexin	Renal	No dose reduction Give 6 hourly	No dose reduction Give 6 hourly	250 mg 12 hourly	Removed by haemodialysis	Give 500 mg after each dialysis
Cefuroxime	Renal	No dose reduction Give 8 hourly	500 mg (adults) 8–12 hourly	500 mg (adults) every 12 hours	Removed by haemodialysis	
Cefazolin	Renal	No dose reduction Give 8 hourly	Reduce dose to 50% 12 hourly	Reduce dose to 25% every 24 hrs	Removed by haemodialysis	
Cefoxitin	Renal	No dose reduction Give 8 hourly	No dose reduction Give 12–24 hourly	Reduce dose to 50% every 24 hrs	Removed by haemodialysis	Give loading dose of 1–2 g after each dialysis
Cefotaxime	Renal	No dose reduction Give 8 hourly	No dose reduction Give 8 hourly	Give initial 1 g dose then 50% of usual dose 8–12 hourly		
Co-trimoxazole	Renal metabolised	No dose reduction Give 12 hourly	Reduce dose to 50% 12 hourly, after 3 days standard dosage	Reduce dose to 50% 24 hourly but avoid if possible unless haemodialysed	Removed by haemodialysis	
Sulphonamides	Renal	No dose reduction Give 6 hourly	Normal dose every 12 hours	Avoid (especially sulphadiazine) because of risk of crystalluria	Removed by haemodialysis	Plasma levels should be monitored if drug is given for more than a few days
Trimethoprim	Renal	No dose reduction Give 12 hourly	No initial dose reduction. After 3 days, reduce to 50% full dosage 12 hourly.	Reduce dose to 50% 12 hourly	Removed by haemodialysis	
Clindamycin	Hepatic (renal)	Unchanged	Unchanged	Reduce dose to 300 mg 8 hourly	Not removed by haemodialysis	

Table 14.1 (*cont'd*)

Guidelines for dosage in renal failure (in management of serious infection, where dosage is critical, therapy should be controlled by measurement of serum antibiotic levels)

Drug	Major elimination routes	GFR > 50 ml/min	GFR10–50 ml/ min	GFR < 10 ml/min	Effect of haemodialysis	Remarks
Metronidazole	Renal Hepatic	Unchanged	No dose reduction Give 12 hourly	No dose reduction Give 24 hourly	Removed by haemodialysis	
Isoniazid	Hepatic (renal)	300 mg (adults) 24 hourly	Reduce dose to 50% 24 hourly	Reduce dose to 50% 24 hourly	Removed by haemodialysis	
Amphotericin B	Non-renal ? metabolised	No dose reduction 24 hourly	No dose reduction 24 hourly	No dose reduction 36–48 hourly	Not removed by haemodialysis	Ineffective for renal parenchyma infection in severe RF
Group III: Major dose adjustments						
Gentamicin Tobramycin Amikacin and other aminoglycosides	Renal	Calculate initial dose using nomogram or consult data sheets. Adjust subsequent doses or intervals according to serum levels.			Removed by haemodialysis	Monitor serum levels in order to determine maintenance dosage
Flucytosine	Renal	No dose reduction 6 hourly	50 mg/kg 12–24 hourly	50 mg/kg 24–48 hourly	Removed by haemodialysis	
Ethambutol	Renal	Calculate initial dose according to body weight and degree of renal impairment (see data sheet). Give 24 hourly Give 24–36 hourly Give 48 hourly			Removed by haemodialysis	

15

Antiviral chemotherapy

Virus replication is so intimately associated with the host cell that it has been very difficult to develop agents which act selectively against viruses, without being unacceptably toxic to mammalian tissue.

INTERFERONS

These are proteins produced by virus-infected cells; they protect other cells from viral infection. Interferon is prepared from human leucocytes and tissue cultures, but until recently it has been difficult and expensive to produce enough for therapeutic evaluation. There has been considerable interest of late in the application of interferon in the treatment of tumours as well as in virus infections.

AMANTADINES

These agents block the entry of virus particles into the host cell. They are active against influenza A and have been used in the prevention of influenza. They shorten the febrile course of the illness by about a day if given early enough, and may be useful for prevention of influenza in institutions caring for the elderly, or those predisposed to serious chest infections; they are relatively non-toxic but occasionally produce neurological disturbance (confusion, vertigo, insomnia).

IDOXURIDINE

A thymidine analogue which inhibits thymidine incorporation in DNA synthesis. It has been used topically in the treatment of *Herpes simplex* keratitis and skin infections. It may accelerate healing of *Herpes zoster* skin lesions if applied early enough. It is very toxic when given systemically and has been superseded by newer agents in treatment of disseminated *Herpes simplex* infection.

VIDARABINE (*Adenine Arabinoside*)

Adenine arabinoside has similar activity to idoxuridine but is somewhat less toxic to bone marrow. It may be used topically for herpes keratitis and systemically for generalized *H. simplex* infections and herpes encephalitis (where treatment must be started as soon as possible) and for chickenpox and *H. zoster* infections in immunocompromised patients. Blood counts should be monitored when the drug is given systemically.

ACYCLOVIR

A guanine derivative absorbed preferentially by herpes-infected cells and selectively phosphorylated by herpes-specified thymidine kinase. The metabolite is much more active against viral than cellular DNA polymerase. *Herpes simplex* is very susceptible although *Herpes varicella/zoster* is less sensitive; activity against cytomegalovirus is variable. It is available for topical treatment of herpes keratitis and genital herpetic lesions. Its toxicity appears to be low and there are good reasons to be optimistic about the application of systemic acyclovir in generalised herpes infections and in oral prophylaxis of such infections in immunocompromised patients. It is now marketed for systemic use specifically for the treatment of *Herpes simplex* infections in immunocompromised patients.

16

Antibiotic policies

At least one-third of patients in hospital receive antibiotics. It is essential that these agents are used in ways which offer the best treatment for individuals, whilst preserving their usefulness in the community by strategies aimed at controlling the emergence of resistance. Widespread use of antibiotics selects resistant strains which readily proliferate if selection pressure of intensive antibiotic use is not relieved. Conversely, a high incidence of antibiotic resistance may be reduced by withdrawal of a heavily prescribed antibiotic.

THE PURPOSE OF HOSPITAL ANTIBIOTIC POLICIES

Control of antibiotic resistance
Bacterial resistance problems reflect antibiotic prescribing habits; the most important function of an antibiotic policy is to foster rational prescribing. Serial passage of organisms in vitro in the presence of antibiotics may induce resistance, and by analogy may occur in hospital wards when bacteria exposed to antibiotics are transferred from patient to patient. Bacteria should be denied this opportunity by careful antibiotic prescribing and control of cross-infection. Antibiotics should be avoided unless bacterial infection is confirmed or highly likely. Prophylactic use must be governed by carefully defined guidelines, since prophylaxis accounts for most over-enthusiastic use of antibiotics (see p. 86).

Control of unnecessary expense
An apparent profusion of new and often expensive drugs is making rational prescribing increasingly complicated; many agents largely duplicate the functions of antibiotics already available and offer little or no advantage over existing drugs. Pharmacies, in collaboration with medical staff, should try to limit stocks of antibiotics routinely available to avoid unnecessary cost incurred by outdated drugs, which may accumulate if too wide a range is kept.

Control of antibiotic toxicity

The policy should reinforce the need to reserve potentially toxic drugs for treatment of infections not susceptible to other antibiotics.

Education

Discussion between clinical staff, medical microbiologists and pharmacists should play an important part in the formulation and application of an antibiotic policy as well as in the treatment of individuals. Periodic review of antibiotic prescriptions and drug resistance patterns should serve as a basis for an active education programme aimed at controlling excessive or irrational use of antimicrobials.

THE FORMULATION OF AN ANTIBIOTIC POLICY

Hospital Drug and Therapeutics Committees should include clinical staff, a medical microbiologist and pharmacist. The policy may take the form of a statement of principles to guide prescribers, reinforced by some limitation in the range of antibiotics purchased and by restricted laboratory reporting of antibiotic sensitivities. More rigid policies may be appropriate in some hospitals where antibiotic resistance is a serious problem; such policies usually involve limiting the prescription of certain antibiotics to senior members of medical staff. For example, antibiotics may be allocated to the following categories:

Antibiotics requiring no restriction

For treatment of sensitive infections or when clinically indicated, this group includes benzylpenicillin, flucloxacillin and other drugs to which resistance is not a problem and which are relatively inexpensive and non-toxic. Hospitals should decide which agents should be allocated to each category, according to local requirements and resistance patterns.

Antibiotics whose use must be restricted

Controlled prescriptions

This group includes valuable drugs to be used carefully in order to preserve the sensitivity of bacteria, e.g. gentamicin, chloramphenicol and parenteral cephalosporins. These drugs should be available on the recommendation of senior members of staff.

Reserved antibiotics

Drugs active against most bacteria, such as amikacin, should be used only for infections not susceptible to other antibiotics. Topical use of antibiotics, except in eye infections, must be carefully controlled. Prescriptions for reserved antibiotics should be endorsed by a consultant's signature.

REVIEW OF THE POLICY

The policy should be reviewed annually in the light of any changes in bacterial resistance or antibiotic use. It is important that information should be effectively disseminated to medical staff if it is to influence prescribing habits.

Further reading

Edwards D (1980) Antimicrobial Drug Action, Macmillan, London

Kucers A, Bennett N M (1979) The Use of Antibiotics, 3rd edn. Heinemann, London

Garrod L P, Lambert H P, O'Grady F (1981) Antibiotic and Chemotherapy, 5th edn. Churchill Livingstone, Edinburgh

Greenwood D (1983) Antimicrobial Chemotherapy, Balliere Tindall, London

Tyrell D A, Phillips I, Goodwin C S, Blowers R (1980) Microbial disease: the use of the laboratory in diagnosis, therapy and control. Edward Arnold, London

Index

Actinomyces israeli, 9
Acyclovir, 98
Amantadine, 97
Aminoglycosides, 41
  mode of action, 5
  (see also individual agents)
Aminoglycoside-inactivating enzymes,
  5, 15
Amoxycillin, 8, 9, 28
Amphotericin B, 68–69
Ampicillin, 8, 9, 27
Antibiotic assays, 89–90
  (see also serum levels of antibiotics)
Antibiotic-associated colitis, 12, 47, 57
Augmentin, 29
Azlocillin, 11, 32

Bacampicillin, 30
Bacillus anthracis, 8
Bactericidal activity of antibiotics, 5, 21
Bactericidal activity of serum during
  antibiotic treatment, 90
Bacteristatic activity of antibiotics, 5, 21
Bacteroides fragilis, 12, 15, 38
Bacteroides spp, 12
Benzylpenicillin, 7, 8, 23
Beta-lactamsases, 3, 15, 29
Beta-lactamases, staphylococcal, 15, 23
Borellia vincenti, 13
Bordetella pertussis, 9, 45
Botulism, 12
Brucella spp, 9, 55

Campylobacter, 11, 45
Candida, 68–72
Capreomycin, 67
Carbenicillin, 30
Carfecillin, 30–31
Cefaclor, 36
Cefamandole, 37
Cefazolin, 36
Cefotaxime, 10, 39
Cefoxitin, 38

Cefsulodin, 40
Ceftazidime, 40
Cefuroxime, 7, 8, 10, 38
Cephalexin, 10, 35
Cephaloridine, 34
Cephalosporins, 34
Cephalothin, 34
Cephradine, 35
Chlamydial infections, 13, 46, 55, 57
Chloramphenicol, 7, 8, 9, 10, 11, 53–54
  mode of action, 5
  acetylases, 15
Chloroquine, 75, 76
Cholera, 55
Cinoxacin, 61
Clavulanate, 29
Clindamycin, 7, 46–47
  mode of action, 5
  resistance to, 16
Clostridium botulinum, 12
Clostridium difficile, 12
Clostridium perfringens, 12
Clostridium tetani, 12
Clotrimazole, 70–71
Cloxacillin, 26
Colistin, 48
Combination antimicrobial therapy,
  21–22, 91
Conjugation, 16
Conjunctivitis (bacterial), 44, 53
Corynebacterium diphtheriae, 8
Co-trimoxazole, 9, 11, 50–51
Coxiella burneti, 13
Cycloserine, 66

Disc tests for antibiotic sensitivities, 90
Doxycycline, 56–57
Diphtheria, 8, 46
  prophylaxis of, 86

Econazole, 71
Empirical antibiotic therapy, 18
Endocarditis, infective, 7, 8, 9, 10, 11,
  26

Entamoeba histolytica, 58
Enterobacter spp, 11
Erythromycin, 7, 8, 11, 45–46
  mode of action, 5
  resistance to, 16
Escherichia coli, 10
Ethambutol, 64–65

Fansidar, 78–79
Flucloxacillin, 6, 26–27
Flucytosine, 69–70
Framycetin, 45
Fungal infections, 68–73
Fusidic acid (sodium fusidate) 47–48
  mode of action, 5
  resistance to, 16

Gardnerella vaginalis, 58
Gas gangrene, 12
Gastro-enteritis, 11
Gentamicin, 8, 10, 11, 41–42
Giardia lamblia, 58
Gonorrhoea, 9, 25, 26, 51, 57
Griseofulvin, 72–73

Haemophilus influenzae, 9, 15, 27, 45, 53
Hepatic failure, antibiotic use in, 92
Herpes simplex, 97, 98
Herpes zoster, 97, 98
Hookworm, 80, 82

Idoxuridine, 97
Interferons, 97
Isoniazid, 62–63

Ketokonazole, 72
Klebsiella spp, 10

Latamoxef, 40
Legionella, 45
Leptospira, 13
Listeria monocytogenes, 8

Malaria,
  treatment of, 74, 76
  prophylaxis of, 76–79
Maloprim, 78
Mebendazole, 80
Mecillinam, 33
Meningitis, 7, 8, 9, 10, 40, 49, 53
Metronidazole, 5, 8, 9
  mode of action, 4
Mezlocillin, 32
Miconazole, 71
Minimum inhibitory concentrations of
  antibiotics, 90
Minocycline, 57

Mycobacterium leprae, 13
Mycobacterium tuberculosis, 13, 62–67
Mycoplasma, 13, 55

Nalidixic acid, 60–61
  mode of action, 4
Neisseria gonorrhoeae, 9, 15, 23, 38, 45
Neisseria meningitidis, 9, 23, 49
Neomycin, 44
Netilmicin 43–44
Niclosamide, 81
Niridazole, 82–83
Nitrofurantoin, 59
Nocardia, 9, 50
Non-specific urethritis, 55
Nystatin, 69

Osteomyelitis, 7, 10, 26, 47, 48
Otitis externa, 44
Oxamniquine, 83

Para-aminosalicylate, 66
Penicillins, (see individual agents) 23
  mode of action, 3
  fixed ratio combination penicillins, 28
Phenoxymethyl penicillin (penicillin V),
  24
Piperacillin, 11, 33
Piperazine, 80
Pivampicillin, 30
Pivmecillinam, 33
Plasmids, 16
Plasmodium falciparum, 74, 75, 76
Plasmodium malariae, 74
Plasmodium ovale, 74
Plasmodium vivax, 74, 75
Pneumocystis carini, 13
Pneumocystis pneumonia,
  Co-trimoxazole in, 51
Polymixins, 48
  mode of action, 4
Praziquantel, 83
Primaquine, 75
Procaine penicillin, 25
Proguanil, 77
Prontosil, 1
Prophylaxis, antimicrobial, of,
  burns, 50
  clostridial gas gangrene, 85
  diphtheria, 86
  endocarditis, 84–85
  malaria, 76–79
  meningococcal meningitis, 85
  recurrent rheumatic fever, 84
  tuberculosis, 63

Prophylaxis, antimicrobial, in surgery, 86–88
  biliary surgery, 87
  colo-rectal surgery, 86–87
  gastric surgery, 87
  hip replacement, 87
  open heart surgery, 87–88
  urological surgery, 88
  vaginal hysterectomy, 87
Proteus spp, 10
Providentia, 11
Pseudomonas spp, 11, 14, 30–33, 39, 40, 41, 48
Psittacosis, 55
Pyrantel, 82
Pyrazinamide 66
Pyrimethamine, 77

Quinine sulphate, 75

R-factors, 16
Renal failure, antibiotic use in, 92–96
Resistance to antibiotics, 14–17
Respiratory tract infections,
  lower respiratory tract, 7, 8, 9, 11, 27, 29, 32, 38, 45, 51, 52
  upper respiratory tract, 7, 8, 9, 25, 27, 29, 45, 51, 52, 55
Rifampicin, 7, 11, 63–64
  mode of action, 4
Ringworm, 70, 71, 72–73
Roundworm, 80

Salmonella typhi, 11, 33
Salmonella (food poisoning serotypes), 11, 33
Salvarsan, 1
Schistosomiasis, 82–83
Selection of antibiotic-resistant bacteria, 15–16
Septicaemia, 7, 8, 9, 10, 11
Septic arthritis 7, 10
Serum levels of antibiotics, (see also antibiotic assays), 89–90
  recommended levels for
  amikacin, 43
  chloramphenicol, 54
  ethambutol, 65
  gentamicin, 42
  streptomycin, 65
  tobramycin, 42
  vancomycin, 57
Shigella sp. 11
Silver sulphadiazine, 50

Soft tissue infections, (including wound sepsis), 7, 8, 14, 25
Spectinomycin, 45
Staphylococci, 23, 41, 47, 63
  Beta-lactamases of, 3
Staphylococci, coagulase-negative, 26
Staphylococcus aureus, 7, 16, 26, 47, 56
  treatment of nasal carriage of 44
Streptococci,
  α- or non-haemolytic, 8
  anaerobic streptococci, 12
  beta-haemolytic streptococci, 7, 26, 27, 55
  Streptococcus faecalis, 8, 22, 27
  Streptococcus pneumoniae, 8, 14, 23, 27, 45
Streptomycin, 44
  resistance to, 16
  in tuberculosis, 65
Strongyloides stercoralis, 81
Sulphonamides, 49
  mode of action, 4
Sulphadiazine, 9, 49, 50, 53
Sulphadimidine, 49, 50
Sulphafurazole, 49, 50
Syphilis, 21
Synergy, between antibiotics, 21

Talampicillin, 30
Tapeworm infestations, 81–82
Tetanus, 12
Tetracyclines (see also minocycline and doxycycline) 10, 11, 54–56
  mode of action, 5
Thiabendazole, 81
Ticarcillin, 31
Tinidazole, 59
Toxoplasma gondi, 13
Transduction, 16
Transmissible resistance, 16
Treponema pallidum, 13, 23
Trichomoniasis, 58
Tuberculosis, 62–67
Typhoid fever, 11, 33, 53

Urinary tract infection, 8, 9, 10, 11, 27, 29, 31, 33, 35, 49, 51, 52, 59, 60, 61

Vancomycin, 8, 57
  mode of action, 4
Vibrio cholerae, 11
Vidarabine, 98
Vincent's angina, 58

Whipworm, 80